60 Seconds to Boost Your BRAIN POWER

60 Seconds to Boost Your BRAIN POWER

The 4-Week Plan to SUPERCHARGE YOUR BRAIN

Michelle Schoffro Cook, PhD, ROHP, DNM

RODALE.

This book is intended as a reference volume only, not as a medical manual.
The information given here is designed to help you make informed decisions about your health.
It is not intended as a substitute for any treatment that may have been prescribed by your doctor.
If you suspect that you have a medical problem, we urge you to seek competent medical help.

Mention of specific companies, organizations, or authorities in this book does not imply
endorsement by the author or publisher, nor does mention of specific companies, organizations,
or authorities imply that they endorse this book, its author, or the publisher.

Internet addresses and telephone numbers given in this book
were accurate at the time it went to press.

© 2016 by Michelle Schoffro Cook

Printed in the United States of America

Rodale Inc. makes every effort to use acid-free ♾, recycled paper ♻.

Book design by Christina Gaugler

"Curried Sweet Potato and Apple Soup" (page 242) and
"Roasted Sweet Potato Salad" (page 249) courtesy of Miriam Rubin;
"Rice Salad with Curried Tofu" (page 254) courtesy of Melissa Lasher;
"Roasted Miso-Ginger Tofu" (page 266), "Green Beans with Walnuts" (page 276), and
"Stir-Fried Asparagus with Sesame Seeds" (page 277) courtesy of Sandra Gluck.

Library of Congress Cataloging-in-Publication Data is on file with the publisher.

ISBN 978–1–62336–465–6 direct hardcover

2 4 6 8 10 9 7 5 3   direct hardcover

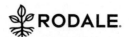

We inspire and enable people to improve their lives and the world around them.
rodalebooks.com

To my wonderful parents, Michael and Deborah Schoffro.
Thank you for your support and love all these years.

To the love of my life and my husband, Curtis Cook.
You make life wonderful. Thank you, always.

CONTENTS

Part I: Build a Better Brain & Memory

Part II: 60-Second Brain Boosters

Part III: Brain-Boosting Recipes

ACKNOWLEDGMENTS

Thank you to my excellent agent and friend, Claire Gerus. Thanks for your vision and the extensive work you do to get my books out there in the hands of readers.

Thank you to Anne Egan, Lora Sickora, and the team at Rodale. I appreciate your continued support of my work and your expertise in editing, design, marketing, and project management, all of which have made *60 Seconds to Boost Your Brain Power* what it is and what it will become.

Thanks to my parents, Michael and Deborah Schoffro, for your ongoing belief in me throughout my lifetime.

Last but definitely not least, thanks to Curtis, my husband and soul mate. There are not sufficient words to thank you for all you do for me.

HOW TO USE THIS BOOK

60 Seconds to Boost Your Brain Power is divided into three parts. In Part I, you'll learn about brain diseases, discover exciting new research that shows we have a tremendous amount of control over our brain health, and explore the 4-Week Brain Health Challenge that will help you boost your brain health and improve your memory. You'll continue to follow the basic tenets listed in Chapter 2 throughout the 4-week challenge and, ideally, for life.

In Part II, you will be introduced to simple 60-Second Brain Health Tips that will help you maximize your brain health with minimal effort. Don't worry: It's not necessary to use all of the 60-second tips, except those found in Chapter 3: Substitute. In other sections, you may need to follow only a handful of the tips provided to achieve excellent results. You can choose to follow more tips if you want to. Just don't stress yourself out trying to do too much, since stress can sabotage your best efforts.

In Part III, you'll discover delicious recipes designed to help you achieve success on the program. Most people are surprised by how easy these recipes are and how delicious they taste. They contain many brain-boosting super-foods and other brain health–building ingredients.

While you may have heard or read that there is little you can do to protect yourself from brain diseases, cutting-edge research proves otherwise. With *60 Seconds to Boost Your Brain Power*, you can empower yourself with the best foods, nutrients, herbs, and lifestyle suggestions to keep your brain functioning optimally for life. Soon after making these simple changes, you'll find that your thinking is clearer, your memory is stronger, and your energy is skyrocketing. You'll find that you actually have a tremendous amount of power to prevent brain diseases.

60 Seconds to Boost Your Brain Power
AT A GLANCE

The Brain Health Plan

In Chapters 1 and 2, you'll learn the Principles of the Brain Health Plan. Follow these basic dietary guidelines and exercises to jump-start your results. This will prime your body for success before you move on to the full 4-Week Brain Health Challenge. The Brain Health Plan eliminates common brain-inflaming offenders and incorporates the foods and habits that are essential to building a better brain.

Week 1 of the Brain Health Challenge: Substitute—Foods to Avoid, and the Foods to Replace Them

In Chapter 3, you will discover the harmful foods and food ingredients that may be damaging your brain. Many of these substances are hidden in common, everyday foods. You will learn how to spot them and why you need to avoid them to maximize your brain power. You'll also learn what foods you can eat to replace any you'll be avoiding. Make all of the recommended substitutions this week because eliminating those substances is essential for results.

Week 2 of the Brain Health Challenge: Boost—Eat More of These Brain-Boosting Superfoods

In Chapter 4, you'll learn about the proven brain-boosting foods and how to include them in your diet. Add as many of these new foods as desired this week, and continue eating them throughout the program to boost brain power and reduce inflammation. Choose at least five of these foods each day.

Week 3 of the Brain Health Challenge: Strategize—Adopt These Tips and Tricks to Boost Your Brain and Memory Power

In Chapter 5, you'll learn about the best scientifically proven brain-boosting strategies. You'll discover the best ways to supercharge your mind, including puzzles, tai chi, meditation, stress reduction, sleep, and more. Choose at least two of these strategies and add them to your daily brain-boosting plan to boost your brain and memory power.

Week 4 of the Brain Health Challenge: Supplement—Use These Supplements to Supercharge Your Brain Health and Memory

In Chapter 6, you'll learn about proven brain-building nutrients, herbs, and other remedies; how to supplement with them; which ones to choose to address your specific issues; and how they can improve your brain health. You will learn about niacin's proven ability to protect against Alzheimer's disease, vitamin B_{12}'s ability to improve memory and reduce memory loss, folate's capacity to reduce your risk of Alzheimer's disease, and more. You'll also discover many other proven memory-enhancing, brain-building, and anti-inflammatory herbs such as sage, periwinkle, ginkgo biloba, and ginger. Don't worry: You don't have to take all the remedies. Choose at least two of the recommended brain-boosting supplements this week, in addition to those recommended in Chapter 2. (If you don't have a brain health disorder and just want excellent brain protection, I usually recommend choosing resveratrol and turmeric. You'll find these on pages 117 and 94, respectively.)

Brain-Boosting Recipes

In Part III, you'll find my favorite brain-boosting recipes. This program is packed with delicious foods and mouthwatering recipes, including Blueberry Pancakes (page 210), Pomegranate Lemonade (page 222), Thai Noodle Salad (page 252), Grilled Salmon with Plum-Blueberry-Grape Salsa (page 279), Strawberry-Chocolate Royale (page 298), and many others. You'll also learn how to stock your brain-power kitchen, build a brain-boosting gourmet salad in minutes, find healthy breakfast options, and even boost your brain health while traveling.

PART I

Build a Better
BRAIN &
MEMORY

CHAPTER 1

YOUR MIRACLE BRAIN

The human brain, then, is the most complicated organization of matter that we know.

ISAAC ASIMOV, FOREWORD TO *THE THREE-POUND UNIVERSE* BY J. HOOPER AND D. TERESI

In our modern, digital age, you may be inclined to think that computers are far superior to the human brain, but you'd be wrong. The human brain is one of the most miraculous things on the planet. It is not only capable of advanced thought processes, but it can also change itself to suit its environment and lifestyle. But I'm getting ahead of myself.

Your brain controls all of your bodily functions, moods, memories, and intellectual processes. Whether your brain is healthy and functioning well determines, to a large degree, your experience of the world and that within your own body. Yet we rarely give this impressive organ a second thought. Unless your memory starts to falter or you develop a nervous system condition, you are likely to neglect this powerful orchestrator of your body and, to a large extent, your life.

For many years, scientists led us to believe that we had little control over our brains and their functioning, and even their health. You may have heard from news reports or through your education that the brain is static: Once you hit a certain age, your brain was finished developing. You couldn't improve your intellectual capacity, since that was largely due to genetics, or so we were told. Worse than that, if you developed a brain disease, there was nothing you could do except hope for some miracle drug to help restore your brain health.

Now we know that these outmoded teachings and beliefs are completely wrong. More and more research shows that we have a tremendous amount of control over our brain capacity and health. What we eat, how we live, how much we challenge ourselves, how stressed we are, and many other factors play significant roles in our overall brain health, cognition, and memory, as well as our moods, resistance to brain diseases, and more. While genetics, of course, plays a role, it is not the be-all and end-all we were originally taught.

The statement "you are what you eat" has never been more apt than when discussing brain health. I would expand the original sentiment to "you are what you eat, learn, and live" to reflect that our lifestyle choices have a significant influence on our short- and long-term brain health. We are in an exciting time, during which brain research is skyrocketing and our knowledge of how to keep our brains healthy and prevent brain disease is climbing sharply, as well. Throughout *60 Seconds to Boost Your Brain Power*, I will share the latest, greatest scientific advances about the brain and memory, along with simple ways you can put the research to work for you in your own life to maximize brain health results.

What if you could transform your life in 60 seconds or less each day? What if you could improve your memory while protecting your brain with simple, all-natural foods, herbs, nutrients, and other remedies that are proven to enhance brain health? That's the promise of *60 Seconds to Boost Your Brain Power*!

Whether you're a jet-setting professional, a working parent juggling multiple jobs, or a busy student, the reality of our hectic world is that few of us have enough time to give our health the attention it deserves. But all of us, no matter how busy, can find 60 seconds a day to transform our brain health and lives. Before we discuss the plan and the 60-Second Brain Health Tips you'll find throughout this book, I'd like to share some personal information about how this book and the program within its pages came to be.

THE ORIGINS OF *60 SECONDS TO BOOST YOUR BRAIN POWER*

More than 20 years ago, I suffered from a traumatic brain injury after being involved in a serious car accident. I partially severed my spinal cord and had other injuries, as well. The car was totally destroyed, except for a small part of the door, which allowed me to get out of the car. Immediately after the accident, I lost most function in my left arm and had a breathing impairment. I began suffering other effects of the brain injury, as well, including severe and steady migraines that became a part of my life for many years. As if that wasn't enough, a couple of years later I slipped and hit my head, resulting in a second traumatic brain injury and the aggravation of many symptoms from the car accident. While many of the accident's effects were immediate, some of the effects of the traumatic brain injury took longer to notice, including memory deficits and depression.

In a desperate effort to alleviate the horrendous pain, breathing impairment, partial paralysis, and other symptoms that consumed so much of my life, I began applying my background in nutrition and herbal medicine, and later in natural medicine and acupuncture. I focused on the best ways to heal from a traumatic brain injury and the food and lifestyle choices that support healthy brain function.

Later, as my health improved, I worked with thousands of patients, including many with brain disorders such as Alzheimer's disease, autism, clinical depression, dementia, Parkinson's disease, traumatic brain injury, and others.

I applied my research and the program I had created for my own health to my patients, as well, with excellent results. Throughout this book, I'll share the discoveries, research, and methods that I have used to treat myself and thousands of clients over the years.

I hope that my experience and knowledge will help you improve your brain health and memory and prevent serious brain diseases. More recently, together with my publisher, Rodale, I developed and conducted a 4-week brain health challenge by applying the program outlined in this book to see if we could get significant memory and brain health results in as little as 4 weeks. The results were impressive. The participants in the 4-Week Brain Health Challenge who made the minimum effort to apply this program to their lives had great results. Throughout this book, I will share some of their stories and experiences on the *60 Seconds to Boost Your Brain Power* program.

One of the most common sentiments I heard from patients and the brain challenge participants was how easy the program is to apply to day-to-day life. Additionally, most people were surprised by how quickly they began to notice results, not just with memory and mental clarity, but also with energy, moods, and weight.

It seems that many people—myself included, at one time—accept memory loss as a part of life. But new scientific research is showing that we will no longer have to accept a declining memory as "just a part of aging." Scientists continuously prove that smart nutrition and a healthy lifestyle go a long way toward protecting your brain and memory from damage.

Before I share the research-based program I developed over more than 22 years, it is valuable to assess your current brain health status. While the best way to fully assess your brain health is through diagnostic tests performed by your doctor, you can also gain insight into your brain health and how your diet and lifestyle choices may be impacting it, either positively or negatively, by completing the brain health assessment on page 10. Of course, if you are suffering from any brain disease or symptoms of a brain

The Facts about Alzheimer's Disease and Parkinson's Disease

You likely know someone, perhaps even a close friend or relative, who has been diagnosed with Alzheimer's disease or Parkinson's disease. Let's take a closer look at these disorders, including the most common symptoms.

Alzheimer's disease is a brain disorder that starts with memory loss and eventually leads to full-blown dementia. There are many symptoms associated with this disease, including memory problems, confusion and disorientation, inability to manage tasks, hallucinations and delusions, episodes of violence and rage, episodes of childlike behavior, paranoia, depression, and mood swings.

Alzheimer's affects a part of the brain called the hippocampus, which is responsible for memory and intellect. Neurons in the hippocampus become entangled, resulting in lost brain cells and abnormal protein fragment formations called plaques or amyloid plaques. Scientists are still unsure whether the tangles and plaque formation cause Alzheimer's disease or whether they are a side effect of the condition. Wherever the plaques are formed in the brain, there is accompanying inflammation, suggesting that inflammation is a factor in the disease.

Parkinson's disease is a disorder of the nervous system that affects movement. The condition develops gradually and usually starts with barely noticeable tremors in one hand. Tremors are the most known sign of the disease, but Parkinson's also causes stiffness or slowing of movement, lack of expression, and slurred speech. While there is no known cure for the disease, diet and lifestyle may help slow the condition and improve quality of life for sufferers.

injury or impaired mental function, you should see your doctor. But even if you've been diagnosed with a brain disease such as Alzheimer's, Parkinson's, dementia, or clinical depression, you will likely find that this plan can help slow, or even potentially reverse, many of the symptoms or even the disease progression. Alternatively, even if you have no signs of a brain disease and simply want to ensure long-term brain health and prevent future brain illness, you will find the program easy to follow and implement in your life.

Signs of a Traumatic Brain Injury

After I slipped and hit my head, I had a headache but no other symptoms to suggest that I might have had a concussion. I went to sleep that night, which is contraindicated with concussions, but I didn't know I had one. The next morning, I awoke and stepped out of bed. I collapsed in a heap when my legs didn't support any weight. I looked sort of like Bambi, the baby deer, first learning to walk. I pulled myself over to the phone and made arrangements to get to a doctor, who assessed me and immediately confirmed that I had a traumatic brain injury. In addition to a possible lack of communication between the brain and limbs, here are some other symptoms of a traumatic brain injury.[1] Keep in mind that the symptoms may vary depending on the severity of the brain injury and the part of the brain injured. It is important to be examined by a doctor as soon as you suspect a traumatic brain injury.

PHYSICAL SYMPTOMS

- Clear fluids draining from the nose or ears
- Convulsions or seizures
- Difficulty sleeping

- Dilation of one or both pupils
- Dizziness or loss of balance
- Excessive sleepiness
- Fatigue or drowsiness

- Inability to awaken from sleep
- Loss of consciousness, for anywhere from a few seconds to a few hours
- Loss of coordination
- Nausea or vomiting

- Persistent headache or a headache that becomes progressively worse
- Weakness or numbness in fingers and toes

SENSORY SYMPTOMS

- Blurred vision
- Ringing in the ears
- A bad taste in the mouth

- Changes to the ability to smell
- Sensitivity to light or sound

COGNITIVE OR MENTAL SYMPTOMS

- Agitation, combativeness, or unusual behavior
- Anxiety
- Coma
- Depression

- Difficulty concentrating
- Memory problems
- A state of severe confusion or disorientation

(continued on page 14)

The Brain Health Assessment

The following brain health assessment can give you a snapshot of your current brain health. It's also a good idea to repeat the assessment at regular intervals after you've completed the 4-Week Brain Health Challenge. You, like many of my brain challenge participants, will likely be surprised by how much your score will improve after only 4 weeks on the plan. And if you retake the quiz regularly, you'll probably notice additional improvements over time, as well. Seeing the change in your score will motivate you to stay on the plan. But experiencing the health benefits—to your brain and overall—is the strongest motivator to continue.

So before we get into the specifics of the program, take the quiz below, which will help you determine your risk of brain disease. Once you total your score, read the results on how the 4-Week Brain Health Challenge can help you.

1. Have you ever been diagnosed with Alzheimer's disease? If yes, ___ score 4 points.

2. Have you ever been diagnosed with Parkinson's disease? If yes, ___ score 4 points.

3. Have you ever been diagnosed with a traumatic brain injury or ___ other brain disease (i.e., ALS [Lou Gehrig's disease], multiple sclerosis, etc.)? If yes, score 4 points.

4. Have you ever been diagnosed (by a doctor) with clinical depres- ___ sion, schizophrenia, bipolar disorder, or another mental health disorder? If yes, score 4 points.

5. Do you have a history of concussions? If yes, score 3 points; give ___ yourself an additional point if you lost consciousness during the concussion.

6. Have you ever been diagnosed with high blood pressure? If yes, ___ score 3 points.

7. Have you ever been diagnosed with heart disease? If yes, score _N_
   3 points.

8. Have you ever been diagnosed with high cholesterol? If yes, _N_
   score 2 points.

9. Do you take statin drugs? If yes, score 3 points. _N_

10. Have you ever been diagnosed with type 2 diabetes? If yes, _N_
    score 3 points.

11. Do you have an immediate family member (parent, brother, or _3_
    sister) who has been diagnosed with Alzheimer's or dementia?
    If yes, score 3 points.

12. Do you have an immediate family member (parent, brother, or _N_
    sister) who has been diagnosed with Parkinson's disease? If yes,
    score 3 points.

13. Do you eat fast food more than once a month? (This includes _N_
    packaged, processed, and commercially prepared foods, use of
    bottled sauces and condiments, and restaurant visits.) If once a
    month, score 1 point; if once a week, score 2 points; if 2+ times
    per week, score 3 points; if daily, score 4 points.

14. How often do you do 30 minutes of cardiovascular exercise? _0_
    (It must raise your heart rate to qualify.) If never, score 4 points;
    if once a month, score 3 points; if once a week, score 2 points;
    if 2 times per week, score 1 point; if 3+ times per week, score
    0 points.

15. Do you work out for more than 2 hours a day, 7 days a week? If _N_
    yes, score 3 points.

16. How many alcoholic beverages do you drink in a week? If you _2_
    drink 1 to 4 alcoholic beverages weekly, score 1 point; if you drink
    5 to 10 alcoholic beverages weekly, score 2 points; if you drink
    11 to 15 alcoholic beverages weekly, score 3 points; if you drink

more than 15 alcoholic beverages weekly, score 4 points. If you don't drink, score 0 points.

17. How much do you smoke? If you have never smoked, score _0_ 0 points; if you smoke less than 1 pack per day, score 3 points; if you smoke more than 1 pack per day, score 4 points; if you quit more than 5 years ago, score 1 point; if you quit less than 5 years ago, score 3 points.

18. How often do you get less than 7 hours of sleep per night? If never, _1_ score 0 points; if less than once a month, score 1 point; if less than once a week, score 2 points; if 2 or more times per week, score 3 points; if every night or almost every night, score 4 points.

19. How often do you drink sugary beverages (such as soda or lattes _3_ with syrup or whipped cream) or sweetened juices or eat sweetened cereals, other sweetened prepared foods, or sweet desserts? If once a month, score 0 points; if once a week, score 1 point; if 2 or 3 times a week, score 2 points; if every day, score 3 points; if more than once a day, score 4 points.

20. How frequently do you try new things (new foods, new courses, _1_ new physical activities, etc.)? If once a month, score 3 points; if once a week, score 2 points; if 2 or 3 times a week, score 1 point; if every day, score 0 points.

21. How often do you learn new, mentally challenging things _0_ (i.e., through reading mentally challenging books; watching educational documentaries; participating in workshops or classroom or distance learning courses; or other mentally challenging activities)? If once a month, score 3 points; if once a week, score 2 points; if every day, score 0 points.

22. Do you feel emotionally supported by your partner, family, or _0_ friends? If "definitely," score 0 points; if "most of the time," score 1 point; if "sometimes," score 2 points; if "rarely," score 3 points; if "never," score 4 points.

23. How positive would other people say you are? Be honest. If _____ 1 extremely, score 0 points; if mostly, score 1 point; if somewhat, score 2 points; if not at all, score 4 points.

Total Score _14_

2/1/02

YOUR SCORE

0 to 10 points
Excellent work! Your score is the brain health version of Mensa status. You're making excellent dietary, lifestyle, and learning choices to keep your brain in tip-top condition. Your risk of brain disease, provided you continue making great choices, is low.

11 to 20 points
Your risk of a brain disease may be low, but you need to make improvements to your diet, lifestyle, and learning choices to ensure your long-term brain health. Take the 4-Week Brain Health Challenge to experience improvements and to set the stage for even better long-term brain health.

21 to 30 points
Now is the time to make diet, lifestyle, and learning changes to lower your risk of brain disease. It's important to reduce low-grade inflammation, give your brain the foods and nutrition it needs, as well as boost your exposure to new ideas and experiences. If you've been sedentary, it's important to start being active. Even just getting up off the couch for a brisk, 30-minute daily walk can give your brain the boost in oxygen that it needs to function properly.

30+ points
Your risk of brain disease is too high, or you've already been diagnosed with one. It's imperative that you give your brain all the foods, supplements, and lifestyle support it needs to function at its peak. Even if you've already been diagnosed with a brain disease or a past traumatic brain injury, you can experience profound improvements in your brain health going forward. There's no time like the present to make the health improvements necessary for your brain health.

NOTE:
Regardless of your score, if you've been diagnosed with a traumatic brain injury or a brain disease such as Alzheimer's or Parkinson's, it is imperative to begin making dietary and lifestyle changes to maximize your brain health and to support your brain with critical nutrients to slow the progression of these diseases.

THE WONDROUS POWER OF YOUR BRAIN

Your brain is truly miraculous. It is constantly changing and regulating billions of different bodily functions at the same time, every second of every day. Your brain orchestrates the complete renewal of your skin every 28 days, your heart every 30 days, and your lungs every 70 days. And these are just a few of your brain's miraculous functions. It also governs your thoughts, moods, emotions, movements, speech, and more.

The average person's brain weighs 3 pounds, yet it has more than 100 billion brain cells, known as neurons. Neurons are connected to each other through synapses, which act like telephone lines between brain cells, carrying information back and forth. If you took all of the phones in the world and all of the phone lines and wires, the trillions of calls daily would not compare to the complexity of the activity within one human brain. The brain is so remarkable that no computer on the planet compares to it, either.

While you may think of your brain as a product of your genes and mostly unchanging, growing until you reach a certain age and then unaffected by your lifestyle and environment, the reality is that your brain is always in a state of change. In addition to all of the functions your brain orchestrates, it has the ability to "clean house" to eliminate connections between brain cells no longer in use. Imagine if your closet could clean itself out, disposing of any clothes you haven't worn in a while and automatically refilling itself with new clothes based on your changing preferences and desires. That's a lot like what your brain can do. Every second of every day your brain assesses the connections between brain cells to determine if they have been used in a while. If they haven't, it dismantles them to make room for new connections. If they are in use, it strengthens these connections for future use.

Every brain cell has a long, wire-like structure called an axon that sends out hormones to generate the electrical charge that allows neurons to communicate. These hormones are transmitters of information, or neurotransmitters, as they are called. There are more than a dozen types of neurotransmitters, each of which performs different functions depending on what message the brain cell is trying to send out. Some neurons turn on functions in your body, while others stop functions from occurring. You may have heard of some neurotransmitters, such as dopamine, serotonin, epinephrine, and norepinephrine. Your brain attempts to keep all of these, and other hormones, balanced to help you feel good and to maintain a state of health. If these hormones become imbalanced, illness or disease can strike, as you'll learn later in this book.

Balanced neurotransmitters aren't the only predictor of brain health; inflammation is also a factor. While many doctors and patients alike don't worry about inflammation of the brain unless it is extremely severe, as in the case of a traumatic brain injury or encephalitis, low-grade, ongoing inflammation can be a real problem for long-term brain health and the prevention of brain disease.

The person who exemplifies the immense potential of the human brain

The Facts about ALS (Lou Gehrig's Disease)

ALS stands for amyotrophic lateral sclerosis. It is a brain disease that causes muscle weakness and impacts physical function. Named "Lou Gehrig's disease" after the famous baseball player who suffered from the disorder, it is a type of motor neuron disease that causes nerve cells to gradually break down. It is also sometimes called motor neuron disease.

Scientists still aren't sure what causes the disease, and it appears that only a small number of cases are genetic. However, recent research links exposure to pesticides, such as the commonly used weed killer Roundup, to the disease,[2] making toxin exposures an important area of future research.

ALS usually begins with muscle twitching, weakness in an arm or leg, and sometimes slurred speed. Over time, it can affect muscular control. While there isn't a known cure, diet and lifestyle may help manage the disease and possibly slow its progression.

is actually an infant. It may seem surprising that an infant's brain best demonstrates everything the human brain offers, but it's true. By about 8 months old, a baby's brain has about 1,000 trillion connections, half of which will die off by the time the child is only 10 years old, leaving 500 trillion to last throughout the rest of his life.

An infant's brain develops faster and better during the first few years of life than at any other time. A young child is constantly absorbing information from sights, sounds, smells, touches, and tastes, as well as through interactions with humans, animals, and other living beings (such as insects, amphibians, and plants). Scientists hypothesize that a baby's brain forms such an enormous number of synapses to ensure that he will have enough "wiring" to receive input from any environment he is born into, as well as to last him his entire lifetime of experiences.

A rich sensory environment is as critical to an infant's development as adequate nutrition. And both are essential throughout a person's lifetime, regardless of his or her age.

Few people recognize the importance of adequate nutrition to the building and maintenance of a healthy brain. Yet your digestive system breaks down every food you eat into nutrients that act as building blocks for every single cell in your body, including all of your brain and nervous system cells. And when the food you eat lacks nutrients, or worse yet, contains harmful sugars, toxic fats, or chemical additives, your brain not only misses the nutrients it requires for health, but it must also deal with the onslaught of harmful ingredients your body was never intended to deal with.

THE BRAIN DISEASE-INFLAMMATION LINK

Scientists have linked chronic, low-grade inflammation with many serious health problems, including arthritis, asthma, heart disease, and cancer. Many now believe that it is also an underlying factor in brain diseases such as depression and possibly dementia.

While the link between brain diseases and inflammation is still in the early stages of investigation, it warrants serious consideration. That's because inflammation is increasingly viewed as an indicator of poor health. Because it is such an important disease predictor, more and more doctors are testing for a marker of inflammation known as C-reactive protein as part of their laboratory testing and investigations into potential causes of ill health.

Inflammation is necessary for survival. It's a clear sign that your immune system has gone into combat mode to fight viruses, bacteria, fungi, or other foreign invaders that may jeopardize your health. When you get a cut or experience an infection, your immune system sends in its frontline defenses in the form of white blood cells and cytokines that can target invaders and send them packing. When that happens, you may experience swelling or feverishness—clear signs of inflammation and an active immune system. While the immune response is necessary for your health and sometimes even for your life, it can sometimes continue after it is no longer needed.

When inflammation lasts for the longer term, or becomes chronic, it can

The Facts about Depression

Everyone feels down at some point in life, usually as a reaction to difficult circumstances; however, clinical depression goes beyond that experience. In clinical depression, the person experiences a prolonged sadness that is out of proportion with the apparent cause. The physical and psychological symptoms affect a person's capacity to function normally in the world.

Depression is often accompanied by sleep disruption, fatigue, anxiety, mood swings, prolonged lapses of concentration, pain, apathy, decreased sex drive, and suicidal thoughts. Because these symptoms can be attributed to other diseases or conditions, it is always important to consult a medical doctor for a diagnosis.

damage your body. Cytokines can stay in your bloodstream and damage tissue. An increasing number of studies show that chronic inflammation in the brain can cause anxiety, fatigue, pain, depression, and other serious health conditions.

A study conducted by Honglei Chen, MD, PhD, and his colleagues at the Harvard School of Public Health found that inflammation plays an important role in the development of Parkinson's disease.[3] Additional research in the journal *Neurology* found that anti-inflammatory approaches seem to prevent and treat the disease.[4] Inflammatory processes also appear during the development of Alzheimer's disease.

In addition to the obvious problem—chronic inflammation in the brain wreaking havoc—there is another problem: We still lack brain imaging devices sensitive enough to pick up most cases of inflammation. That's why increasing numbers of health practitioners are testing for C-reactive protein, since it is a clear marker for inflammation in the body and/or brain.

How to you get this Test

While we wait for the science to catch up, engaging in a diet and lifestyle that quell inflammation is an effective way to address the problem at its source. That's where *60 Seconds to Boost Your Brain Power* comes in. It is based on research-proven foods, strategies, lifestyle changes, and nutritional and botanical medicines that reduce inflammation and prevent or reverse brain disease.

The program also works to reduce stress, which is a well-established trigger of inflammation. Research even links a difficult childhood to higher rates of chronic inflammation, making it important for people who experienced stressful childhoods to get on top of the inflammation that may be behind their brain health issues. In a study of nearly 1,000 people ages 45 to 90 with cardiovascular disease, those who experienced major stressors, such as natural disasters or serious car accidents, had higher levels of inflammation in their bodies.[5] Other research links stress early in life to higher rates of inflammatory diseases in adulthood.[6]

More than 100 studies show that environmental, nutritional, and lifestyle

The Facts about Huntington's Disease

Huntington's disease (HD) is a serious degenerative brain disorder that affects muscles, memory, and behavior patterns of people suffering from the illness. HD is an inherited brain disorder that causes cells in parts of the brain to prematurely die, specifically in the caudate, the putamen, and, as the disease progresses, the cerebral cortex. As the brain cells die, a person with HD becomes less able to control movements, recall events, make decisions, and control emotions.

factors play a significant role in initiating or accelerating brain disease. Fortunately, the program outlined in this book works to address the stress, inflammation, and environmental, nutritional, and lifestyle factors that are linked to brain health and disease. In the next chapter, we'll further explore the nutritional way to significantly reduce inflammation in your body.

HOW TO TRANSFORM YOUR BRAIN

No longer do you need to stand idly by, hoping that you will avoid the ravages of memory loss, dementia, or brain disease. By following the program outlined in this book, you can make simple changes to your diet, lifestyle, and daily routine that will result in a supercharged memory, resilience against brain disease, and superior brain health. *60 Seconds to Boost Your Brain Power* offers the principles of the Brain Health Plan along with simple dietary and lifestyle changes that take less than 60 seconds each and result in a stronger mind and brain. You will discover the foods, strategies, and supplements that can have your brain healthier than ever.

We all know that heart disease and cancer are our two primary killers; these diseases will take the lives of a record number of North Americans. But there's an even greater threat that will overshadow both of these in deadly impact: According to new research, scientists predict that within 8 years, brain diseases will kill or disable more North Americans than cancer and heart disease combined! That means a huge number of people need help protecting and healing their brains.

With *60 Seconds to Boost Your Brain Power*, you can feel confident that you are taking charge of your brain health. You will no longer have to accept a declining memory as "just a part of aging." Scientists continuously prove that smart nutrition and a healthy lifestyle will protect your brain and memory from damage and can even aid in the prevention of serious brain diseases, including Alzheimer's and Parkinson's.

Though the blood–brain barrier was once believed to be impermeable, we now know it works through a lock-and-key mechanism. Damaging chemicals can mimic vital nutrients and gain access to your brain, where they can cause inflammation and plaque. Unfortunately, many of these toxins are commonly found in our foods, homes, and offices.

But this book is about empowerment and health. With a minimum amount of effort, you can employ the knowledge you gain to lock out neurotoxins, quell inflammation in your brain, and fortify this essential organ with proven brain-protecting nutrients and phytonutrients (plant nutrients). It's all about boosting your brain health and improving your memory right now. This book is for anyone who cares about his or her brain. That means everyone!

You'll discover my solid plan for building a better brain, along with a research-proven holistic approach and a practical way to ensure that you can easily adapt it to your life. I will guide you through the foods to swap, foods to eat, natural remedies that can supercharge your brain, and strategies to boost your memory. Each week you'll replace foods in your diet with better options, make minor adjustments to your lifestyle, or add remedies that build brain power.

I'll also reveal how you can balance your brain neurotransmitters, strengthen your memory (only one of your brain's many functions), shield your brain from neurotoxins (substances proven to damage your brain and nervous system), and fortify your brain against inflammation or disease. Plus, this book is packed with research-supported, cutting-edge tips that will help you build a better brain 60 seconds at a time.

You will find 60 brain-boosting tips in *60 Seconds to Boost Your Brain Power*. Additionally, every brain booster in this book offers a Super Health Bonus, which is featured at the end of each tip. With this program, you'll supercharge your brain health and, at the same time, energize your body, improve your immunity to illness, and restore your youthful appearance! I'm not aware of any drugs that offer these impressive health benefits as side effects, but the best brain-building foods, nutrients, herbs, and lifestyle strategies ensure that you'll protect and boost your brain while feeling better than ever in every aspect of your life. So let's move on to the next chapter, where I'll share the fundamentals of the Brain Health Plan so you can begin to reap the amazing health rewards immediately.

CHAPTER 2

BUILD A BETTER BRAIN

It is unmatched in its ability to think, to communicate, and to reason. Most striking of all, it has a unique awareness of its identity and of its place in space and time. Welcome to the human brain, the cathedral of complexity.

PETER COVENEY AND ROGER HIGHFIELD, *FRONTIERS OF COMPLEXITY*

Let's discuss the Principles of the 4-Week Brain Health Challenge so you can get started eliminating brain-inflaming offenders and build a better brain through your food and lifestyle choices. This chapter provides the first layer of lifestyle and dietary advice you will follow over the next 4 weeks—or for as long as you'd like. Keep in mind that the more you incorporate these suggestions throughout your life, the more likely it is that you'll maintain a healthy brain for life.

I call these the Principles because they are the basis for your brain health program. This practical, step-by-step, anti-inflammatory brain health plan will help you transform your potentially brain-harming diet into a much healthier, brain-supporting one.

Once you feel comfortable with the information presented in this chapter and you've started making the recommended changes to your diet and lifestyle, you can start to add the 60-Second Brain Health Tips that begin in the following chapter.

Keep in mind that we'll be exploring different foods and strategies in greater detail as we progress. In this chapter, I'll explain the research and rationale behind each part of the plan, so don't worry if you're feeling confused or a bit overwhelmed at first. It will all make sense by the end of this chapter.

I recommend adding the tips one week at a time. For example, once you're accustomed to the Principles of the 4-Week Brain Health Challenge and the 60-second tips in Chapter 3: Substitute, the following week, add five of the "Boost" foods from Chapter 4 that build brain health, and so on until you've added tips from each of the four following chapters.

While the 4-Week Brain Health Challenge is designed to be implemented over 28 days (jumping into Week 1 at the same time as you begin following the Principles), it's okay to spend a week or more getting used to the Principles of the 4-Week Brain Health Challenge before starting the tips in Week 1. You can also spend additional weeks adjusting to each new phase, if you prefer. In this way, you can customize the plan to your particular needs and move at your preferred pace, which will help you make lasting changes.

THE INFLAMMATORY STANDARD AMERICAN DIET

Let's face it: Most Americans love sitting down to a hearty breakfast of bacon, eggs, and coffee, perhaps with some milk and sugar added. Or perhaps a dinner of steak and potatoes, white pasta with cream sauce, and a decadent dessert is more your speed? Yet these and many other everyday foods are linked to low-grade inflammation. That might not sound like a big deal, but when you consider that brain diseases have been linked to inflammation, it is imperative to address the inflammation as part of our 4-Week Brain Health Challenge to ensure brain health for life. Let's briefly explore some of the worst problems with the Standard American Diet to demonstrate how we may be unintentionally weakening our brain health through the foods we choose.

Bad Fats and Wrong Fats, Oh My

Your brain is 60 percent fat and needs plenty of high-quality dietary fat to create healthy brain cells. Getting sufficient amounts of brain-building fats is one of the best things you can do for your brain. Yet most people ingest trans fats (found in packaged, prepared, and fast foods, as well as many baked goods and restaurant foods), which can actually damage your brain by creating inflammation in your brain and body. Shortening and margarine and anything in which they are found are also sources of unhealthy trans fats. That includes baked goods, cookies, pies, and buns. Of course there are healthier alternatives to these baked goods, but they're hard to find because most grocery stores and bakeries are using these harmful ingredients. Trans fats have even been found to damage the protective blood–brain barrier required to keep your brain healthy, thereby allowing harmful substances access to your delicate gray matter.

It's not just these harmful fats that create a problem for the brain and the blood–brain barrier. You've probably heard about beneficial omega-3 fatty acids, as they have been getting a lot of attention in the media. There are also beneficial omega-6 fatty acids, but most people get more of the latter fats than they need. Actually, most people eat 20 to 40 times as many omega-6 fatty acids as they do omega-3 fatty acids. While omega-6 fatty acids are beneficial to your health in moderate amounts, in this ratio, they cause excessive inflammation. Omega-3s are needed in sufficient amounts to keep the inflammation at bay, yet most of us don't get enough of these critical fats.

The Standard American Diet contains few, if any, omega-3 essential fats. These critical nutrients are needed to protect your brain from inflammation and to maintain healthy brain cells and signals between them. Our diet tends to be higher in omega-6s, or worse, trans fats. Corn, safflower, and sunflower oils, as well as the ambiguous "vegetable oil" commonly used in most North American households and restaurants, are all sources of omega-6s. (Vegetable oil is often used to fry food or as an ingredient in bottled sauces, mayonnaise, and other prepared foods.) Omega-6s are also found in meat from animals that eat foods high in omega-6s, such as those mentioned above. Our heavy consumption of these foods plays a role in the distorted ratio of omega-6s to omega-3s.

Omega-3s are found in flaxseeds and flaxseed oil; chia seeds; canola, olive, and walnut oil; dark, leafy greens, such as spinach and kale; and fatty fish, such as wild salmon, mackerel, sardines, anchovies, and others.

It's not just the warped ratio of essential fatty acids that predisposes us to inflammation and a deficit of healthy fats to replenish brain cells, it is also the quality of the oils we eat. All oils have different smoke points—the temperature above which the oil begins to smoke and is no longer healthy to eat. When oils smoke, their delicate essential oils become damaged, cause inflammation, and in some cases also become carcinogenic. Because of this, oils that have extremely low smoke points, such as flaxseed oil, should never be heated. Olive oil smokes at just under 325°F, while macadamia nut oil reaches its smoke point around 410°F. Most oils sold in grocery stores, however, have been heated to extremely high temperatures during their processing and packaging, even before you get them home and begin to cook with them. These overheated or rancid oils no longer support brain health and actually create inflammation. Extra-virgin olive oil is the exception. Some grocery stores are moving to refrigerated, cold-pressed virgin oils, but this is still fairly rare. Most health food stores offer healthier, refrigerated, cold-pressed oils.

I probably don't need to explain that fried foods such as French fries, onion rings, potato chips, and nachos cause inflammation. I think these items speak for themselves. Most of us know that fried foods, which are highly inflammatory in the body, have no redeeming health quality. That's because the oils tend to be heated to excessive temperatures and are used over and over again. When oils are heated past their smoke point or are reused on a frequent basis, they become inflammation-causing oils.

You'll learn more about these harmful fats and how to replace them with healthier options in 60-Second Brain Health Tip #4 on page 57.

Good Carbs, Bad Carbs

Fats aren't the only problem in your diet. Your brain also requires adequate energy to fuel its many functions. While energy can come from multiple dietary sources, foods that contain complex carbohydrates are the primary source. Yet most people eat the wrong kinds of carbs and insufficient amounts of the good carbs that fuel the brain, leaving it with insufficient energy to perform its vital tasks.

Your brain needs a slow and steady supply of energy to ensure that it always has fuel to function properly. Imagine how poorly your car would function if you tried to give it the wrong fuel, or if you overfilled the gas tank and then went for long periods of time during which you neglected to give it any gas at all.

But this is exactly what we do with our brains. You may give yours refined sugars from pastries, doughnuts, candy, cakes, white bread, white rice, and white potatoes instead of the correct fuel from legumes, vegetables, and certain whole grains that break down slowly and steadily. You may gorge on sugary foods that cause your blood sugar to quickly surge and then plummet within an hour or two, meaning that your brain won't have the fuel it needs and leaving you feeling forgetful, exhausted, moody, depressed, or craving sweets. Or you may skip breakfast, wait long periods between meals, or eat at irregular times. All of these bad habits mean that your brain won't have sufficient energy to accomplish its functions at optimal levels. And you may be left wondering why you feel so terrible, why your memory is so bad, or why you are irritable.

12 Surprising Sources of Hidden Sugar

Sugar hides in many unexpected places. Considering that sugar consumption has been linked to many illnesses and that even a few teaspoons of sugar will shut down your immune system for up to 6 hours, it is important to be on the lookout for sugar. Be sure to read labels to identify ingredients that end in "-ose," such as glucose, maltose, fructose, high fructose corn syrup, etc. All of these ingredients are sugar in its myriad forms. Additionally, there are many ways that sugar can sneak into your diet, even if it does not appear on the label. Here are 12 surprising sources of hidden sugar identified in Nancy Appleton's book *Lick the Sugar Habit:*[1]

- The breading on most packaged and restaurant foods contains sugar.

- Sugar (in the form of corn syrup and dehydrated molasses) is often added to hamburgers sold in restaurants to reduce meat shrinkage during cooking.

- Before salmon is canned, it is often glazed with a sugar solution.

It is important to significantly reduce your consumption of sugar, sweets, soft drinks, and sweetened juices. Research shows that sugar is one of the most addictive substances you can use. It's also highly inflammatory. No, you don't need to eliminate sugar and sweets altogether; simply reduce your consumption and make fruit your go-to food when you're craving something sweet. You'll learn more about the damaging effects of sugar and how to replace it with healthier options in 60-Second Brain Health Tip #1 on page 49.

I probably don't need to go into much additional detail about the wrong carbs, since most of us know that the sweets we eat aren't good for us. What you may not realize, however, is how much sugar hides in surprising places.

- Many meat packers feed sugar to animals prior to slaughter to "improve" the flavor and color of cured meat.

- Some fast-food restaurants sell poultry that has been injected with a sugar or honey solution.

- Some table and seasoning salts contain sugar!

- Sugar is used in the processing of luncheon meats, bacon, and canned meats.

- Most bouillon cubes contain sugar (and usually MSG, as well).

- Peanut butter tends to contain sugar.

- Dry cereals often contain high amounts of sugar.

- Almost half of the calories in commercial ketchup come from sugar.

- More than 90 percent of the calories in a can of cranberry sauce come from sugar.

Eating the wrong types of fats in unhealthy ratios, insufficient brain-building fats, and excessive amounts of sugar are just a couple of dietary habits that contribute to memory problems and, in some cases, even brain diseases.

A Drink Is Just a Drink?

Alcoholic beverages such as beer, spirits, and wine act similarly to concentrated sugar in your body and are best eliminated or used in moderation. While there's a lot of hype about red wine's ability to boost brain health, this belief is largely based on the notion that the benefits of the resveratrol found in red wine outweigh the brain-cell-killing effects of the alcohol it contains. I'll explain more about resveratrol and better ways to obtain this brain-boosting nutrient in 60-Second Brain Health Tip #28 on page 117. Of course, that doesn't mean that you need to give up alcohol completely, but it's best not to drink it every day.

Sugar by Any Other Name

You may be thinking that synthetic sweeteners might be a good alternative to sugar, but they are actually worse than sugar. There are many different types of artificial sweeteners, including NutraSweet, Splenda, saccharin, aspartame, and AminoSweet, but they are all best avoided due to their negative health effects. Research links these nasty substances to many serious health conditions, from headaches and depression to Parkinson's-type symptoms. I avoid them like the plague, and I think you'll want to, too, after you read more about these nasties in Brain Health Principle #9 on page 41.

The Meat of the Matter

Red meat and antibiotic- and hormone-laced poultry are well-established causes of inflammation in the body. I'm not suggesting that you have to go vegan or vegetarian here (although a plant-based diet tends to be much lower in inflammatory substances), but meat and poultry tend to cause inflammation, so make them the background of your meals—not the main dish. Simply reducing the amount of meat in your diet and selecting hormone- and antibiotic-free poultry will go a long way toward reducing inflammation. Wild-caught fish tends to be high in omega-3 fatty acids and is anti-inflammatory, making it an excellent choice. You will also learn more about the importance of reducing your meat consumption and great high-protein vegetarian options in 60-Second Brain Health Tip #5 on page 59.

The "3 Ps"—Processed, Packaged, or Prepared Foods

Most processed, packaged, and prepared foods top the list of inflammatory foods thanks to their harmful oils, sugar and artificial sweeteners, additives, and a whole host of nasty ingredients. There are many different artificial ingredients found in these foods, all of which are best avoided: colors, flavor enhancers, stabilizers, preservatives, etc. (Some of the main ones include sulfites, benzoates, and colors named FD&C # "X.") Of course, a package of legumes or quinoa is not the same as the vast majority of fast-food and prepared food items to which I'm referring. It's a good idea to read package labels to see if they contain any of these untoward ingredients. Keep in mind that most fast foods and prepared foods made in-house at grocery stores will not have ingredients labels, but I guarantee that almost all of these items are packed with potentially neurotoxic (damaging to nerve and brain cells) ingredients and are best avoided. By reducing your consumption of processed, packaged, and prepared foods, you'll go a long way toward eliminating harmful food additives from your diet.

Milk Myths and Dairy Dangers

Got milk? If so, you might want to rethink your decision to eat dairy products. While dairy marketing boards spend millions to convince us that we need milk for a healthy body, there are many reasons to avoid dairy products such as milk, yogurt, ice cream, cottage cheese, butter, and cheese. Dairy products cause inflammation in your body. Some of the reasons dairy products are inflammatory are linked with current ranching, manufacturing, and commercialization practices. Today's dairy products differ greatly from those made even a century ago. Now they contain hormones, antibiotics, and other harmful ingredients, so they are best avoided as much as possible, unless you're choosing organic options. But even organic dairy causes inflammation in many people.

Dairy product consumption has even been linked to an increased risk of Parkinson's disease, according to a meta-analysis study published in the *European Journal of Epidemiology*. According to the research, the more dairy consumed by study participants, the greater their likelihood of experiencing Parkinson's. The risk of Parkinson's increased by 17 percent for every 7 ounces of milk consumed per day. In other words, the more milk people drank, the greater their risk.[2] Don't forget that milk is an ingredient in many baked goods, pastries, breads, and beverages and is found in other unexpected foods, as well.

Here are several more reasons why it is best to eliminate or significantly reduce your dairy intake.

1. Cow's milk is intended for baby cows. We're the only species (other than those we domesticate) that drinks milk after infancy. And we're definitely the only species drinking the milk of a different species. Baby cows have four stomachs to digest milk. We have one.

2. Dairy products contain hormones. Not only are the naturally present hormones in cow's milk stronger than human hormones, the animals are routinely given steroids and other hormones to plump them up and increase their milk production. These hormones can negatively impact your delicate human hormonal balance.

3. Most cows are fed inappropriate food. Commercial feed for cows contains all sorts of ingredients, including genetically modified corn, genetically modified soy, animal products, chicken manure, cottonseed, pesticides, and antibiotics. Can you guess what that feed becomes? The milk you drink.

4. Research shows that the countries whose citizens consume the most dairy products have the highest incidence of osteoporosis, contrary to what dairy bureaus try to tell us.

5. Research links dairy products with the formation of arthritis. In one study of rabbits, scientist Richard Panush was able to produce

inflammation in the joints of animals simply by switching their water to cow's milk. In another study, scientists observed more than a 50 percent reduction in the pain and swelling of arthritis when participants eliminated milk and dairy products from their diets.[3]

6. Most dairy products are pasteurized to kill potentially harmful bacteria. During the pasteurization process, vitamins, proteins, and enzymes are also destroyed. Enzymes assist with the digestion process, and when these enzymes are destroyed, the milk becomes harder to digest, which puts a strain on your body's enzyme systems.

7. Most milk is homogenized, which denatures the milk's proteins, making it harder to digest. Many people's bodies react to these proteins as though they are "foreign invaders," causing their immune systems to overreact, which ultimately results in inflammation.

8. Pesticides in cow feed find their way into the milk and dairy products that you consume. Pesticides are neurotoxins that can be harmful to your body.

The Whole Grain and Nothing But the Grain

White flour bread, pastries, and other baked goods are best avoided altogether during the 4-Week Brain Health Challenge. That's because white flour acts the same way as sugar in your body and is replete with all the problems of sugar that you learned about earlier in this chapter. And while many people think that whole wheat products are health foods, they aren't. Many whole wheat breads, pastas, and pastries contain white flour along with a small amount of whole wheat flour or a multigrain mix. Both white flour and whole wheat flour, and therefore the products made with them, tend to be inflammatory in your body once eaten.

Additionally, some people react to the gluten these products contain. Gluten is a particular type of protein found in some grains and is highly inflammatory

Prescription Meds Linked to Brain Diseases

There is a silent brain disease culprit that few people know about: prescription medications. Some medications have been linked with symptoms of brain diseases, and worse, brain diseases themselves, so it is imperative to check the prescriptions you're taking if you are experiencing any memory or cognitive problems. Some prescription medications may be mimicking brain diseases or actually causing brain diseases such as Alzheimer's. New research in the *British Medical Journal* shows that there are strong ties between some popular medications—namely a class of drugs called benzodiazepines (BZDs)—and dementia. The main culprits are antianxiety and insomnia medications such as diazepam (Valium) and alprazolam (Xanax), both of which are BZDs, since research has found that taking these drugs more than doubles a person's risk of Alzheimer's disease.[4]

Other smaller-scale studies had already identified a possible benzodiazepine–dementia link, but the *BMJ* study strongly supports the connection. And while discontinuing these drugs is a good place to start (with the help of your doctor, of course), the study found that

to some, but not all, people. If you have unexplained health problems for which your doctor can find no cause, or you have many seemingly diverse health issues, I recommend a visit to a naturally minded health practitioner who can test you to determine whether you have a gluten allergy or sensitivity. Additionally, there are many grains and grain product alternatives that do not contain gluten and are delicious. You can also switch to these gluten-free alternatives to see if you experience improvements. Keep in mind that if you have a gluten sensitivity or a full-blown allergy, it is imperative that you eliminate gluten altogether. Even cheating once in a while will negate any benefits of eating gluten-free the rest of the time. Also, keep in mind that while gluten can be extremely having taken these drugs for 3 months or longer at some point in the past increases your risk for Alzheimer's disease by 51 percent compared to people who were never prescribed BZDs. According to the study results, the longer a person used BZDs, the higher their risk of Alzheimer's. While international drug guidelines for BZD use call for their short-term use only (less than 3 months), many people, under the guidance or neglect of their physicians, have used these medications for much longer periods.

If you choose to stop taking these brain-damaging drugs, and I believe that is the best option for most people, it is important to work with your physician, because quitting them cold turkey can lead to potentially scary symptoms, including panic attacks, headaches, and even suicidal thoughts. Your doctor can help to gradually wean you off the medication, thereby avoiding uncomfortable or serious withdrawal symptoms.

While you will experience brain health benefits from this program even if you're taking these drugs, obviously the results will be superior if you remove serious obstacles to brain health, such as BZDs.

dangerous for some people, it is not something that needs to be entirely avoided by most people. If you don't have a gluten allergy or sensitivity, simply reducing the number of gluten-containing foods in your diet goes a long way toward reducing inflammation.

In addition to white flour and whole wheat flour, other gluten-containing grains to reduce your consumption of (or avoid altogether, if you are allergic) include rye, spelt, kamut, and some oats and oatmeal. If the label on the oats or oatmeal does not say that it contains "gluten-free" oats, then the product probably contains gluten. Try reducing your consumption of these gluten-containing foods as much as possible, with the goal of significantly reducing or eliminating them completely. Instead, choose gluten-free grains or seeds such as buckwheat, quinoa, millet, brown rice, wild rice, and black rice (also called forbidden rice), and use the flours made from them for baking.

THE PRINCIPLES OF THE 4-WEEK BRAIN HEALTH CHALLENGE

Let's get to work building a strong and healthy brain that is resilient against brain diseases, memory loss, and cognitive impairment. Even if you've already started experiencing a serious brain disease, you can benefit from following the principles of the 4-Week Brain Health Challenge. To build a sensational brain, you need to eat a diet that is high in brain-building nutrients, including amino acids found in protein, healthy sugars found in healthy complex carbohydrates, and essential fatty acids found in healthy fats, as well as a mix of vitamins and minerals. When you eat a healthy, brain-building diet like the one I outline here, your body will break down the foods into these components, which act as the building blocks of a healthy brain.

Brain Health Principle #1: Cut back on red meat and dairy products. As you've already learned, red meat and dairy products contain saturated fats that tend to increase blood cholesterol levels and encourage your body's production of beta-amyloid plaques in your brain, increasing your risk of brain diseases such as Alzheimer's. In the Chicago Health and Aging Study, people who consumed the highest amounts of saturated fat had three times the risk of developing Alzheimer's disease.[5] Eat no more than one serving of meat or dairy products (½ cup of dairy or 6 ounces of meat) no more than five times weekly. On the days you avoid red meat, you can eat up to 6 ounces of lean poultry or fish. Ideally, you should be having a couple of vegetarian days a week, as well. Some people already occasionally have "meatless Mondays," and if you're among them, you're halfway there.

Amino acids are the building blocks of protein. When you eat protein-rich foods, your body breaks them down into amino acids and other nutrients that your brain cells can use. While amino acids are required by your brain for optimal health, you need to be sure that your body is able to break down the protein foods to extract those amino acids, and from this standpoint, not all protein-rich foods are created equally. While meat and poultry are fine in small amounts, most people eat far too much of these foods, and that contributes to excess amounts of omega-6 fatty acids, and worse, excessive amounts of saturated fats that break down into inflammatory arachidonic acid. As you learned earlier, omega-6s are fine when consumed in a healthy ratio to omega-3s, but most people eat excessive amounts that contribute to inflammation. Similarly, saturated fats are healthy and safe in small amounts, but the amount most people eat exceeds the upper limit.

Some foods that are high in digestible and highly usable protein include avocados, legumes such as lentils or kidney beans, nuts, nut butters, almond milk, soy milk, tofu, bean sprouts, and alfalfa sprouts. Also, when bean sprouts are eaten raw, they are loaded with highly absorbable protein thanks to enzymes they contain that allow for quick-and-easy digestion. You'll learn more about plant-based sources of protein in 60-Second Brain Health Tip #5 on page 59.

We need to stop equating "protein" with "meat." Thanks to the high-protein diet craze, I get so many people asking how they will get adequate protein in their diets—even though I counsel that most foods contain protein, and many vegetarian sources of protein are actually superior, due to their digestibility.

Brain Health Principle #2: Avoid refined grains and enjoy whole grains, instead. Emphasize gluten-free options like quinoa, brown rice, millet, wild rice, amaranth, teff, tapioca, arrowroot, and sorghum.

Your body breaks down healthy carbs into the natural sugars that your brain needs for its energy supply. I can almost hear some readers justifying their sugar addictions with that statement. However, your body has specific sugar needs. Refined or concentrated sugars, such as those found in sodas, ice cream, cakes, cookies, or other sugary foods, provide a quick sugar rush that just as quickly causes blood sugar levels to plummet. That kind of sugar roller coaster is detrimental to your brain health, not to mention your immune system.

Instead, your brain requires sustained energy from healthy carbs such as fruits, whole grains, and legumes. Legumes are high in both protein and carbs, making them an excellent food choice for brain health.

As you learned earlier, many grains contain gluten, a sticky substance that causes an immune response in gluten-sensitive individuals. Like other sensitivities, gluten sensitivity rarely causes the same symptoms as pollen and environmental allergies. Instead, gluten may contribute to low-grade inflammation throughout your body. Since inflammation is linked to many brain diseases, it is best to avoid gluten-containing grains as much as possible. The main ones include wheat (which includes whole wheat and white flour, as well as anything made with them), rye, kamut, and spelt.

According to archaeological evidence, humans didn't start eating grains until the onset of the Agricultural Revolution about 10,000 years ago. Prior to that, we subsisted largely on fruits, nuts, seeds, wild vegetables, herbs, and possibly some meat, although experts differ in their opinions. Some experts believe that this is why so many people have difficulty handling many grains, particularly those containing gluten. While we'd like to think of our bodies as adapting quickly, when it comes to their nutritional needs and digestive capacities, they don't.

Additionally, it is important to choose whole grains over refined grains. Refined grains cause rapid blood sugar fluctuations that are linked to energy deficits in the brain, as well as inflammation. Dana Carpender, author of *500 Low-Carb Recipes*, once told me in a private interview, "Enriched-flour products are typically grain products that have had all the fiber and some 35 or more nutrients removed and 5 added back in. Enriched-flour products are comparable to being robbed of all your clothes, money, shoes, and personal belongings while walking to the bus stop. Then the thief gives you your shoes and a quarter for the bus and tells you that you've been 'enriched' by the experience. Not likely."

Better sources of gluten-free whole grains and carbohydrates include brown rice, wild rice, black rice, almond flour, tapioca flour, amaranth, arrowroot, and quinoa. Brown rice is more nutritious and a better option than white rice. It offers vitamin E and is high in fiber. Quinoa, a staple of the ancient Incas who revered it as sacred, is not a true grain, but rather a seed. It is a complete protein and is high in iron, B vitamins, and fiber. Amaranth is an ancient grain that is packed with important nutrients and devoid of gluten.

Not a true grain, wild rice is actually a type of aquatic grass seed native to the United States and Canada. It tends to be a bit pricier than other grains, but its high content of protein and its nutty flavor make wild rice worth every penny. It is an excellent choice for people with celiac disease or who have gluten or wheat sensitivities. Add wild rice to soups, stews, salads, and pilafs. It is important to note that wild rice is black. There are many blends of white and wild rice, most of which tend to consist primarily of refined white rice. Be sure to use only wild rice, not the blends, to avoid refined rice.

Brain Health Principle #3: Go gluten-free if you are experiencing depression or another mental illness. A recent study in the journal *Biological Psychiatry* found that gluten sensitivity and celiac disease may be linked to schizophrenia and psychosis. Scientists at the Department of Pediatrics at Johns Hopkins School of Medicine studied 471 people, including 129 with recently developed psychosis, 191 with mild schizophrenia, and 151 with neither condition to act as controls for the experiment.

The scientists measured levels of various types of antibodies to determine whether people with either schizophrenia or psychosis had any greater sensitivity to gluten than people without mental illness. Less than 1 percent of those with mental illness showed signs of celiac disease—a disease characterized by an inability to digest gluten and many resulting disabling symptoms. However, a significant number of people with schizophrenia and psychosis had high levels of antibodies to gluten.

The people with mental illness exhibited many of the same symptoms as people with celiac disease, but they had a different immune response. Those with mental illness also differed substantially in their reactions to gluten compared to the control group without mental illness. This study suggests that an abnormal immune response to gluten may be involved with these forms of mental illness. Of course, further research is needed, but this study gives people an important dietary factor to consider when dealing with mental illness.

Brain Health Principle #4: Eat three square meals and snacks. Be sure to eat at least three meals daily with healthy snacks in between to help keep your blood sugar levels stable. Blood sugar is the fuel your brain requires for optimal performance. And it needs a slow and steady supply, which is the exact opposite of the way most people eat: skipping meals, lots of sugar or sweets at certain times of day, and lots of sugar highs and crashes. The best part of eating three meals and a couple of snacks every day is that you don't have to count calories, grams of protein, or other information! As long as you follow the guidelines in this book, you're all set.

Brain Health Principle #5: Eliminate trans fats, hydrogenated fats, and all foods that contain them (margarine, shortening, pastries, biscuits, etc.). Completely avoid all products that contain trans fats or hydrogenated fats. Stanford-trained research scientist J. Robert Hatherill, PhD, found that diets containing trans fats make brain cell membranes excessively permeable, allowing viruses greater access to the brain, disrupting brain signals, causing brain cells to become dysfunctional, and promoting cognitive decline. As if that wasn't bad enough, trans fats also incorporate themselves into the myelin sheath—the protective coating of nerves and brain cells. This changes the electrical conductivity of nerve and brain cells, thereby negatively affecting the body's communications. Trans fats have also been shown to increase the risk of stroke (and heart disease, too).[6]

Brain Health Principle #6: Vegetables and fruits should make up at least 80 percent of your diet. Vegetables should make up the bulk of it. Sorry, white potatoes don't count. Try to incorporate a wide variety of different vegetables and fruits, such as squash, leafy greens, peppers, cabbage, onions, sweet potatoes, apples, pomegranates, cherries, and blueberries. Get at least five servings of vegetables daily. One serving equals approximately ½ cup of each vegetable. Get at least two servings of fruit daily. One serving of fruit equals approximately ½ cup of each fruit, or one fruit with a pit. Be sure to include at least three of the essential brain-boosting foods each day. They include blueberries, grapes, pomegranates, tomatoes, walnuts, and wild salmon. While many of the best brain boosters are fruits and vegetables, other foods belong on this list as well, as you can see from the inclusion of walnuts and wild salmon. Additionally, choose at least two of the other great brain boosters each day. They include apricots, peaches, plums, celery and celery seeds, cherries, coffee, ginger, kidney beans, sage, rosemary, and tea.

Brain Health Principle #7: Switch to coconut oil or extra-virgin olive oil for cooking and baking. That means no canola, vegetable oil, shortening, margarine, etc. While coconut oil contains saturated fats, a growing body of research shows that these saturated facts act differently in your body than saturated fats from animal products, such as meat and dairy.

Brain Health Principle #8: Eat at least ½ cup of legumes daily. You can choose whichever kind you like best: chickpeas, black beans, kidney beans, navy beans, lentils, peas, etc. Only count legumes in which the fiber is still intact—whole beans. That means soy milk and tofu don't count, because the fiber has been removed from these foods. Of course, you can still eat these foods, just don't count them toward your daily legume intake.

Brain Health Principle #9: Avoid artificial sweeteners such as sucralose, aspartame, and saccharin. Choose only stevia or whole food sweeteners (raisins, dates, applesauce, etc.) to sweeten recipes. Keep sugars of all kinds to a minimum. Splenda is also known as sucralose, and while it is advertised as a natural sweetener, it isn't. According to Joseph Mercola, DO, it "has been altered to the point that it's actually closer to DDT and Agent Orange than to sugar."[7] Aspartame also goes by the names AminoSweet and Neotame and has been linked to brain cancer.[8] Saccharin, a coal tar derivative, is also known as Sweet'N Low, Sweet Twin, and Necta Sweet and is considered a "probable carcinogen."[9]

Brain Health Principle #10: Significantly reduce your sugar intake.

Cut back on sweets of all kinds: cookies, cakes, pastries, etc. If you crave something sweet, opt for fruit. If you experience depression or another mental illness, do your best to avoid concentrated sugars altogether. Fruit is fine in moderation.

Brain Health Principle #11: Choose unrefined sea salt over iodized salt. Instead of iodized salt, choose unrefined or Celtic sea salt. Iodized salt is sodium with iodine added, while unrefined sea salt naturally contains sodium along with many other valuable minerals, including potassium, calcium, and magnesium. While salt is never a great source of these types of minerals, unrefined or Celtic sea salt also has many trace minerals that, as their name suggests, your body needs in trace amounts. Iodized salt has none of these trace minerals. Therefore, it is best to choose unrefined sea salt that naturally contains many different minerals, not just sodium and iodine.

Brain Health Principle #12: Get 30 minutes of brisk exercise at least five times a week. Brisk walking, running, hiking, cycling, inline skating, or any other brisk activity is fine. Exercise is critical to ensure that healthy, oxygen-rich blood is delivered in adequate quantities to your brain. A total loss of oxygen for 6 minutes can result in permanent damage to your brain, and 7 minutes can result in death. Because you obtain oxygen through breathing, simply breathing shallowly or not getting sufficient exercise can reduce the amount of oxygen-rich blood that pumps to your brain. By exercising regularly, you'll boost that supply. You'll find some excellent ideas and suggestions in Chapter 5, including 60-Second Brain Health Tips #40 and #42, beginning on page 148.

Brain Health Principle #13: Take a high-quality multivitamin and mineral supplement. It should be free of iron, copper, sugar, additives, colors, and artificial sweeteners. Consume iron supplements only if your physician has instructed you to do so. Make sure your multivitamin contains at least 50 grams of B-complex vitamins and 50 micrograms of folate and B_{12}. Studies link a vitamin B_{12} deficiency to an increased risk of Alzheimer's disease, memory loss, and depression. Research also shows that simply getting more B vitamins (such as from a multiple plus extra vitamin B_{12}) can halve the rate of brain shrinkage associated with aging.[10]

Brain Health Principle #14: Add 60-Second Brain Health Tips. The 60-second tips you'll find in the next part of this book are a critical component of the 4-Week Brain Health Challenge. Don't worry—you don't need to do all of them. Simply include the number of tips recommended at the start of each section. You'll add all of the tips in Chapter 3: Substitute (page 47), five of the foods in Chapter 4: Boost (page 81), two of the lifestyle recommendations in Chapter 5: Strategize (page 127), and two of the natural supplements in Chapter 6: Supplement (page 159). The supplements outlined in Chapter 6 have proven benefits for specific brain diseases, so if you have a specific condition, read through that chapter and choose the supplements suggested for that condition. For example, if you have dementia, choose the supplements suggested for dementia.

But what if you don't have a brain disease and simply want to prevent one? For a good general brain health plan, supplement with curcumin and resveratrol. Supplement with a standardized extract of 1,200 milligrams of curcumin daily and 250 milligrams of resveratrol daily. Ginkgo biloba is an excellent herb for general brain health. Take 120 milligrams of ginkgo biloba daily. Be sure to obtain your physician's approval prior to taking these supplements to ensure that other medications you take won't interact with them. You can take these supplements in divided doses throughout the day, if you prefer. Most people find them easiest to take with a meal or snack.

The Principles of the 4-Week Brain Health Challenge are easy to follow, and the plan becomes easier and easier as you adjust to making better choices and replacing unhealthy foods with delicious and nutritious choices. Throughout this book, I'll discuss more dietary and lifestyle problems and the quick fixes you can make. You'll be shocked to learn about some of the common places brain-damaging chemicals lurk, as well as the impressive foods, herbs, nutrients, and even medicinal mushrooms that hold the greatest promise for the prevention and treatment of brain diseases.

PART II

60-Second
BRAIN
BOOSTERS

CHAPTER 3

WEEK 1: SUBSTITUTE

Foods to Avoid and the Foods to Replace Them

This week I will introduce you to the harmful foods, household products, and ingredients that may be affecting your memory and brain health. Many of these substances are found in common, everyday places. You learned about some of them in the previous chapter, but in this chapter you'll learn how to spot them, why you should avoid them, and how minimizing your exposure to them can significantly improve your brain health. And, of course, you'll learn simple substitutions you can make so you won't miss your favorite foods or products. Follow all of the tips in this chapter for the best brain health benefits.

In this section, you'll learn to:

60-SECOND BRAIN HEALTH TIP #1:
Make the Switch to Stevia

Discover the brain health–friendly sweetener that prevents blood sugar fluctuations and weight gain.

If I told you that there is a white powdery substance that is extremely damaging to your brain, you probably wouldn't think I was talking about sugar. But shocking new research from the School of Medical Sciences at the University of New South Wales, Australia, found that eating a high-sugar diet for just 1 week is enough to cause memory impairment and brain inflammation. According to the lead scientist, Margaret Morris, "What is so surprising about this research is the speed with which the deterioration of the cognition occurred."[1]

If you think this research doesn't apply to you, consider that the Standard American Diet is a high-sugar diet. According to the USDA, the average person eats 156 pounds of added sugar every year. And that doesn't include naturally present sugars in foods such as fruit. Compare that with our ancestors' diets a century ago: They ate only about 5 pounds of sugar each year.

In this excessive amount, sugar is linked to inflammation throughout the body, including the brain. Excessive sugar consumption is linked with a decline in mental capacity and an increase in alpha, delta, and theta brain waves, which alters your mind's ability to think clearly. It has also been linked to learning disorders, poor memory formation, and depression.[2]

Other research shows that a diet high in added sugar reduces the production of a brain chemical known as brain-derived neurotrophic factor (BDNF). Without sufficient BDNF, your brain can't form new memories, nor can you learn new things or remember much. Levels of BDNF are especially low in people with impaired sugar metabolism, such as diabetics and prediabetics.[3] Low levels of BDNF are also linked to depression and dementia. While more research needs to happen to determine whether BDNF is a causal factor in brain diseases such as Alzheimer's, it's already clear that low BDNF is bad for your brain. By taming your sugar intake, you'll help make BDNF your new BFF.

While sugar in its most natural form is fuel for your brain, it is important not to confuse the naturally present sugars in fruits and starchy foods with the refined and concentrated added sugars in much of our processed and prepared foods. There's a big difference. Your brain needs some sugar to function, just like your car needs gasoline to function. But your brain needs the naturally occurring sugars in a slow, steady dose—as happens when you metabolize fruits or starches—not the sugar rushes that come with adding sugar to most of our foods.

Soda is one of the worst sources of sugar, containing 7 to 11 teaspoons per can and much more than that in the supersize beverages now sold at many fast-food places. Sugar is insidious in our diet, hiding in many unsuspected places, including condiments, meat, French fries, and even in some table and seasoning salts. It's shocking but true.

Stevia, or *Stevia rebaudiana,* is a natural herb that tastes sweet but doesn't actually contain sugar molecules. As a result, it doesn't affect blood sugar levels or cause inflammation in the body, and it is therefore a healthy option for a healthy brain. It is naturally between 300 and 1,000 times sweeter than sugar, depending on whether you're using the whole herb or the liquid extract. I personally find liquid stevia to have the best taste and least aftertaste, but I've found powdered versions that are excellent, as well.

How to Benefit

Switch from sugar to the naturally sweet herb stevia. Sugar hides in many packaged and prepared foods. Look for any ingredient name that contains "-ose," such as glucose, high fructose corn syrup, fructose, dextrose, maltose, etc. Even natural sweeteners like honey, pure maple syrup, agave nectar, and barley malt are high in sugars and should be used sparingly. While stevia is available in many forms, be aware that some manufacturers of the powdered extract of stevia include other sweeteners with the herb, so these products are best avoided.

Because stevia is naturally sweet, you won't need much to sweeten your tea, coffee, or other foods and beverages. Just a few drops of the liquid sweeten coffee or tea, and the powder usually comes with what looks like a doll-size spoon because one scoop that size is all you'll need for most beverages.

Baking with stevia poses some challenges because it doesn't have the same chemical properties as sugar, so it doesn't caramelize when heated or become chewy in cookies. Also, because you use so little stevia, it may throw off the traditional dry-to-wet ingredients ratio in some recipes. You may need to experiment a bit with your recipes.

Super Health Bonus

Sugar consumption has been linked to high blood pressure, high cholesterol, heart disease, weight gain, diabetes, and premature aging, to name just a few conditions. By switching to stevia, you'll naturally reduce your risk of experiencing any of these diseases and will slow your aging process. What's more, because even a few teaspoons of sugar can depress your immune system for 4 to 6 hours, you'll probably notice you suffer from fewer colds, flus, and infections after reducing the sugar in your diet.

60-SECOND BRAIN HEALTH TIP #2:
Pass on the Aspartame-Laden Foods and Beverages

Eliminate the artificial sweetener that has been linked to brain tumors and other brain health issues.

Before you take another sip of that aspartame-laden diet soda or other "diet" food or beverage, here are seven brain health reasons to rethink that drink.

1. Only 1 year after aspartame was approved by the FDA, its own task force learned that some of the original data showcasing aspartame's safety had been falsified to hide results showing that animals fed aspartame had experienced seizures and developed brain tumors.[4] The artificial sweetener was never recalled. Aspartame has also been linked to the formation of various types of cancer, including brain cancer.

2. There is a 43 percent increased risk of experiencing a stroke or heart attack when a person drinks more than one diet soda daily.

3. According to the authors of the book *Hard to Swallow,* when a diet drink containing aspartame is stored at 85°F for a week or longer, "There is no aspartame left in the soft drinks, just the components it breaks down into, like formaldehyde, formic acid, and diketopiperazine, a chemical that can cause brain tumors. All of these substances are known to be toxic to humans."[5]

4. According to researchers at the American Academy of Neurology, if you drink four or more cans of soda daily, you're 30 percent more likely to suffer from depression.[6]

5. Research shows that aspartame in diet soda causes an imbalance in brain hormones, specifically dopamine and serotonin.[7] Dopamine is a brain chemical that helps us feel good. Impaired dopamine production is involved in brain disorders such as Parkinson's disease. Serotonin is a feel-good brain neurotransmitter that reduces pain and the likelihood of experiencing depression.[8] Low levels of serotonin have been linked with aggressive behavior.[9]

6. Mold inhibitors added to diet soda cause severe cell damage, according to research by Peter Piper, professor of molecular biology and biotechnology at the University of Sheffield in the United Kingdom. This cell damage likely includes brain and nerve cells.[10]

7. Diet soda as a mix for alcoholic beverages worsens hangovers. According to research at the Royal Adelaide Hospital in Australia, diet soda increases the rate at which alcohol enters the bloodstream and causes hangovers to occur sooner than they otherwise would, as well as making them more intense.[11] The increased rate of alcohol entering the bloodstream can also increase the rate at which brain cells are destroyed.

How to Benefit

If you absolutely must have soda, choose a stevia-sweetened one instead of the many aspartame-laden sodas on the market. One good choice is Zevia. Most "diet" foods and products contain aspartame or other types of artificial sweeteners, so they are best left at the store. Choose unsweetened foods and beverages, and add a few drops of the naturally sweet herbal extract stevia, which you learned about in the previous brain health tip.

Super Health Bonus

It's ironic, considering its name and reputation as a "diet" drink, that diet soda is more likely to make a person fat. It is linked to a 34 percent increase in metabolic syndrome, along with its symptoms of high cholesterol and abdominal obesity.[12] Just drinking two cans of diet soda daily has been linked to a 500 percent increase in waist size.[13] By skipping aspartame, you're likely to lose weight if you're overweight. And since a Harvard University study found that drinking diet soda daily doubles a person's risk of kidney disease, you'll have a reduced incidence of kidney disease, as well.[14] You'll even maintain stronger teeth, since diet soda is extremely acidic and has been linked to dental enamel erosion.[15]

60-SECOND BRAIN HEALTH TIP #3:
Remove the Brain Toxin MSG

Eliminate the food additive that excites brain and nerve cells until they die.

MSG by any other name would still be as harmful. When most people hear the name monosodium glutamate, or MSG, they immediately think of Chinese food. And while the chemical is used in many Chinese food restaurants, this brain and nervous system toxin masquerades under many different guises and even within many food additives.

Considering that MSG has been linked to many serious health conditions, including hormonal imbalances, weight gain, brain damage, obesity, headaches, and more, you may be shocked to learn how prevalent it is. MSG is almost always found in processed, prepared, and packaged foods. Even when there is no sign of it on the label, it is still frequently hidden in many prepared foods.

What's even more shocking is how MSG affects your brain. As you learned earlier, there is a protective mechanism in your brain known as the blood–brain barrier. Your brain depends on careful control of chemicals to operate smoothly. Even small fluctuations in the concentrations of these chemicals can cause drastic disruptions in brain function. When excitotoxins enter your brain, they literally excite brain cells until they die. MSG is added to foods as a taste enhancer, but it is well established in research as an excitotoxin.

Additionally, some parts of your brain, such as the hypothalamus and the pineal gland, are not protected by the blood–brain barrier, yet these parts of your brain control many hormones in your body, as well as other bodily functions, including mood regulation.

When MSG enters your brain, not only does it kill brain cells, but it also wreaks havoc on brain functions. Some research has even linked it to the progression of Parkinson's disease.[16] According to Dr. Patricia Fitzgerald, a homeopath and the author of *The Detox Solution*, "ingesting MSG over the years has also been linked with Parkinson's and Alzheimer's."[17]

Many people react within 48 hours of ingesting even minute amounts of MSG, which can make it difficult to trace back to the food source that caused the reaction. The effects can include headaches, hives, canker sores, runny nose, insomnia, seizures, mood swings, panic attacks, heart palpitations and other heart irregularities, nausea, numbness, asthma attacks, and migraines. Many of my clients also report experiencing restless leg syndrome after accidental ingestion of MSG.

Research shows that MSG enters the brain slowly, bypasses the blood–brain barrier, and reaches peak concentrations in the brain 3 hours after it's ingested. Levels of MSG in the brain remain high for 24 hours after the initial ingestion of the contaminated food.[18] MSG can be especially detrimental to people who have experienced some sort of brain injury or who have a genetic predisposition to brain disease. According to board-certified neurosurgeon Russell Blaylock, MD, long-time MSG researcher and author of *Excitotoxins*, "There is some recent evidence that Parkinson's patients have a defect in their metabolism that leads to increased metabolism. Such a defect would make them more vulnerable to the harmful effects of excitotoxins." MSG is one of the most common excitotoxins to which we are frequently exposed due to its omnipresence in our processed food supply. The artificial sweetener aspartame is also one of the worst excitotoxins. See page 51 for more information about aspartame.

According to Dr. Blaylock, there are many names for this harmful toxin that you should look for on food labels.[19]

ADDITIVES THAT ALWAYS CONTAIN MSG:

- Monosodium glutamate (that's the full name for MSG)
- Hydrolyzed vegetable protein
- Hydrolyzed protein
- Hydrolyzed plant protein
- Plant protein extract
- Sodium caseinate
- Calcium caseinate
- Yeast extract
- Textured protein
- Autolyzed yeast
- Hydrolyzed oat flour

ADDITIVES THAT FREQUENTLY CONTAIN MSG:

- Malt extract
- Malt flavoring
- Bouillon
- Broth
- Stock
- Flavoring
- Natural flavoring
- Natural beef or chicken flavoring
- Seasoning
- Spices

ADDITIVES THAT SOMETIMES CONTAIN MSG:

- Carrageenan
- Enzymes
- Soy protein concentrate
- Soy protein isolate
- Whey protein isolate

How to Benefit

Avoid prepared and packaged foods as much as possible. Also, try to avoid eating at fast-food restaurants, because they are notorious culprits when it comes to MSG usage. If you must buy packaged or prepared foods, be sure to take the above list with you so you can avoid harmful neurotoxins that could be affecting your health. If the product doesn't come with an ingredients list, such as items made in-house at the bakery and deli department in your grocery store, you should assume it contains MSG, as these types of food items frequently do. Avoiding these types of foods will help you reduce your exposure to MSG, but there are also some lesser-known food sources of this harmful chemical. Some of the many culprits include:

Baby food. Shocking as it is, baby food manufacturers often include glutamate, one of MSG's many guises, as a flavor "enhancer."

Bottled sauces. Just gotta have your Thai, teriyaki, or Jamaican jerk sauce? Well, most bottled sauces contain MSG.

Infant formula. As terrible as it sounds, most popular brands of infant formula actually contain MSG in one of its myriad disguises.

Protein powder. Many of the protein powders used for weight loss or muscle building, even those sold in health food stores, contain MSG, usually as hydrolyzed protein or hydrolyzed soy protein.

Croutons. Most croutons are flavored with bouillon, soup base, or "natural" or artificial flavors that contain MSG.

Salad dressings. The salad dressing you choose could negate any of the health benefits of eating salad if you choose a bottled dressing that contains MSG. Bottled salad dressings may contain "natural flavor," "spices," or "seasoning," all of which can legally contain MSG.

Soups. Most soups, even most homemade soups, contain MSG (even if the cook swears they don't). That's because most soup bases, commercial stocks, and bouillon powder and cubes contain MSG. And few nutritionists and even fewer chefs are familiar with MSG's many names.

Soy "meat" products. Many vegetarian burgers, hot dogs, sausages, and other meat alternatives contain textured vegetable protein, hydrolyzed vegetable protein, or hydrolyzed plant protein, all of which usually contain MSG.

Spice mixtures. Love that Cajun seasoning, Tex-Mex rub, or other spice mixture? Most spice mixtures contain MSG—frequently as autolyzed yeast or yeast extract.

Vaccines. Foods are not the only places you're exposed to MSG. You'll probably be surprised to learn that MSG is found in vaccines as a "stabilizer." The chickenpox vaccine made by Merck pharmaceutical company is a primary example. Merck's measles, mumps, and rubella vaccine also contains this harmful neurotoxin.

Super Health Bonus

Because MSG is linked with so many uncomfortable, or even downright dangerous, health symptoms, eliminating it from your diet typically results in fewer headaches, migraines, asthma attacks, and panic attacks. And any sufferer of these conditions knows that reducing them means a much greater quality of life.

60-SECOND BRAIN HEALTH TIP #4:
Replace Trans Fats with Brain-Healthy Choices

Switch from fats that cause brain inflammation to ones that protect your brain from damage.

Trans fats are harmful to every cell in your body, and especially to your brain. They do not occur naturally, but rather are made in laboratories and manufacturing plants in which these oils are heavily processed. This processing involves adding hydrogen atoms to a healthy fat to saturate the fat molecule, thereby turning unsaturated oil into saturated oil. The result is a hydrogenated fat, or trans fat—a type of fat that your body was never intended to ingest or digest. These fats are industrial creations made to extend the shelf life of fats without regard for the effect on human health. Even a few generations ago our ancestors were never exposed to these brain toxins.

Here's why exposure to these fats, found in many of the foods you eat, are a threat to your brain: Trans fats are incorporated into cellular membranes, including brain and nerve cell membranes, by standing in for healthy fats. The result is impaired brain cells. Brain cell membranes need to be pliable to allow their fluid-like properties to function properly. Research shows that molecules of linoleic acid (one type of fat) are more than three times wider than the chemically altered trans fat form of linoleic acid. As a result, researchers speculate that the blood–brain barrier will leak if it is made up of trans fats, which could allow greater quantities of toxins to access your brain than if it were made of healthy fats.

Stanford-trained research scientist J. Robert Hatherill, PhD, made an important discovery about trans fats: Ingesting them makes brain cell membranes excessively permeable. This poses a serious problem, because it means viruses and toxins can gain greater access to your brain, disrupt brain signals, and even cause brain cells to become dysfunctional. Over time, this serious threat to brain health can result in cognitive decline. He also found that brain cell membranes made up of trans fats may increase aluminum uptake into the brains of older individuals.

And if that's not bad enough, what's worse is that people who are deficient in omega-3 fatty acids will absorb up to twice as many trans fats when they eat them, making their brains even more vulnerable to these fats. You'll learn more about brain-healthy omega-3 fatty acids and why most people are deficient in these essential healers in 60-Second Brain Health Tips #22 and #23 on pages 107 and 109.

If you think you're not eating trans fats or hydrogenated fats, here's just a sampling of the places they lurk: margarine, crackers, cookies, pies, vegetable shortening, snack foods, prepared and packaged salad dressings, doughnuts, and French fries, as well as most restaurant foods. For many years, margarine has been billed as a healthy alternative to butter, but many brands of margarine contain trans fats or rancid fats that are best left behind. Margarine is cheap to make, so many manufacturers have profited from the misleading marketing.

And if you think, "Well, I read the packages of the foods I eat and they always say '0 grams trans fats,' so this doesn't apply to me," you're wrong. That's because small amounts of trans fats are allowable in most foods, provided the foods contain less than 1 gram per serving. But when you add up these hidden trans fats, they still spell damage to your delicate brain cells.

How to Benefit

Switching from cookies, crackers, pies, French fries, and snack foods that contain trans fats to ones made with healthier oils will go a long way toward improving your brain and mental health. Better yet, reduce your consumption of these less-than-healthy foods. It's easy to bake French fries that have been made with olive oil rather than eat trans fat–laden ones out of a package or at a fast-food restaurant. Try eating more homemade food without any margarine or other sources of trans fats. I provide an excellent recipe for Brain-Boosting Butter (and it is certainly better than margarine, too) on page 230.

Super Health Bonus

Trans fats cause inflammation, which has been linked to many serious health conditions, including arthritis, cancer, diabetes, and heart disease. If you make a conscious effort to avoid trans fats, your whole body will thank you in the form of a reduced likelihood of these severe conditions.

60-SECOND BRAIN HEALTH TIP #5:

Reduce Meat Consumption to Reduce Inflammation

Simply reducing your intake of meat will help to reduce brain-damaging inflammation.

The link between meat consumption and inflammation isn't exactly news to most people, but it's always great when research backs up our understanding: Eating more meat spells higher inflammation levels in your body.

That's the conclusion of scientists at the Department of Nutrition and Food Sciences, Nutritional Epidemiology, at the University of Bonn in Germany. They examined 46 studies to assess markers of inflammation, focusing on a substance known as C-reactive protein. Other research has shown C-reactive protein to be a precursor to serious, chronic diseases such as heart disease.

In the Bonn, Germany, study published in the journal *Nutrition Reviews*, scientists found higher levels of inflammation markers, especially C-reactive protein, in meat-based or "Western-like" diets, while plant-based diets high in fruits and vegetables tended to result in lower inflammation levels.[20]

That's good news for anyone striving to eat a plant-based diet focused on more fruits and vegetables. Fruits and vegetables are nutritional powerhouses, thanks to their macronutrient content, which includes amino acids, natural sugars for energy, and fatty acids, as well as their micronutrient content, which includes vitamins and minerals. But that's not all. Fruits and vegetables are high in phytonutrients. ("Phyto" means "plant," so "phytonutrients" simply means plant nutrients.) There are hundreds of different phytonutrients in fruits and vegetables, including anthocyanins, carotenoids, catechins, flavonoids, and polyphenols.

Research has shown that phytonutrients help protect your memory, ward off the effects of aging, fight cancer, keep you fitter, and much more. So it's no surprise that a diet high in phytonutrient-rich foods reduces inflammation in your body and brain.

This is good news because inflammation is increasingly being linked to most forms of chronic disease, including heart disease, cancer, diabetes, arthritis, and many others. Knowing that a simple switch to a plant-based diet high in fruits and vegetables can cause a significant drop in disease-producing inflammation means that you can empower yourself to take charge of your health and dramatically reduce your likelihood of experiencing serious illness. If you're already experiencing one of these serious illnesses, then you can empower yourself to take charge of the illness in a natural way, free of side effects.

How to Benefit

It's easy to eat more plant foods. If you're worrying about getting enough protein, consider that the average American eats 248 pounds of meat every year, or about 40 percent of his or her total caloric intake. Most experts agree that no more than 10 percent of our total calories should be obtained from meat. But if you're still concerned, here are some of the best vegan sources of protein.

- Avocado
- Coconut
- Dairy alternatives, including almond milk, coconut milk, hemp seed milk, and soy milk
- Legumes, such as kidney beans, black beans, navy beans, pinto beans, Romano beans, chickpeas, soybeans, and edamame (green soybeans)
- Nuts (preferably raw and unsalted), including almonds, Brazil nuts, cashews, macadamia nuts, pecans, pistachios, and walnuts
- Quinoa
- Seeds, including chia seeds, flaxseeds, hemp seeds, pumpkin seeds, sunflower seeds, and sesame seeds
- Soy products (organic only, since soy is heavily genetically modified), including tofu, miso, and tempeh

You may notice that protein powders are not on the list. That's because many are heavily processed, sugar-laden, or contain monosodium glutamate (MSG) in one of its many guises, particularly protein "isolates." MSG is a well-documented nerve and brain cell toxin that actually stimulates brain cells to death. It's a much better idea to use ground seeds to add protein to your smoothies than it is to use protein powders.

Super Health Bonus

There are many health benefits of eating less meat. The increase in fiber in your diet helps ward off colon cancer, and the ramped-up phytonutrient intake helps prevent heart disease, most types of cancer, and diabetes.

60-SECOND BRAIN HEALTH TIP #6:
Remove Heavy Metals from Your Life

Discover the surprising everyday sources of brain-toxic heavy metals.

When you think of metals, you might think of pots and pans, cars and trucks, or the structural beams for your home, but the last thing you'd probably consider is metals in your brain. And when it comes to metals, the last place you want them is in your brain.

Heavy metal is a serious threat to the health of your body and brain. I'm not referring to Ozzy Osbourne or Metallica here, although too much head-banging has probably damaged more than a few brain cells. I'm referring to the metals found in food, water, air, and many commercially available products. Here are some common metals and their surprising sources:

Aluminum. Although not strictly a *heavy* metal, aluminum can pose a threat to health, particularly with excessive exposure. While the research is still controversial, aluminum has been linked to Alzheimer's disease and Parkinson's disease. It is found in:

- Baby formulas
- Baked goods and processed foods
- Deodorants
- Over-the-counter and prescription antacids (see 60-Second Brain Health Tip #7 on page 65)
- Other pharmaceutical drugs (as a binding agent)
- Aluminum pots and pans
- Shampoos
- Skin creams

Cadmium. This has serious repercussions for your brain and inhibits your body's ability to use nutrients such as iron, zinc, and calcium, leaving you more vulnerable to bone and immune system disorders. Cadmium is found in:

- Automobile seat covers
- Black rubber
- Burned motor oil
- Ceramics
- Cigarettes
- Evaporated milk
- Fertilizers
- Floor coverings
- Fungicides
- Furniture
- Refined wheat flour (white flour)
- Silver polish
- Soft drinks from vending machines with cadmium in the pipes

Copper. While your body needs copper in small amounts to ensure bone growth, nerve function, and tissue formation, researchers at the University of Rochester Medical Center found that copper may be involved in triggering the onset of Alzheimer's disease. According to Rashid Deane, PhD, lead author of the study, excessive copper seems to prevent the brain from getting rid of a protein that forms plaque, which triggers the disease. The study, published in the *Proceedings of the National Academy of Sciences*, showed that copper can also cause the protective blood–brain barrier to break down in animals.[21] There's still controversy over copper's role in brain diseases, particularly since some scientists find that it may have a protective role in the brain. Either way, it's probably safe to say that most of us are getting sufficient copper from our water and diet and should not seek out supplements that contain the mineral. Copper is found in:

- Water in houses or offices supplied by copper pipes
- Some nutritional supplements

- Red meat
- Shellfish

Lead. Linked to dementia, Alzheimer's disease, learning disabilities, seizure disorders, aggression, hyperactivity, and many other health issues, lead is found in:

- Canned foods
- Cigarette smoke (first- or secondhand)
- Colored, glossy newsprint
- Some ceramic dishes
- Lead paint (found in older homes)
- Lead water pipes (found in older buildings)
- Refined chocolate (chocolate that is mostly sugar, dairy, or artificial flavors)
- Vehicle emissions (Even though lead gasoline was banned 3 decades ago in many countries, it has found its way into groundwater, soil, and other places.)

Mercury. Known for its speedy ability to cross the blood–brain barrier, mercury is linked to neurological, psychological, and immunological disorders in people, including diseases like Alzheimer's. It has also been linked to heart arrhythmias, headaches, blurred vision, and weakness. It is found in:

- Silver-looking dental fillings (Many dentists cite studies that show no mercury particles are released from fillings, but numerous studies show that mercury is primarily released as a vapor that gains access to the brain and blood.)
- Fish (Not all fish, but many farmed varieties tend to be contaminated.)
- Immunizations (Many vaccines, even those used for children, contain the mercury-based preservative thimerosal in amounts that are excessive for both children and adults.)

How to Benefit

Iron and steel manufacturing distributes cadmium into the environment and our water supply, but an inexpensive water filter can remove the brain-damaging heavy metal in only seconds. Drs. Richard Casdorph and Morton Walker, leading researchers on heavy metals, insist that changing the disposal requirements for cadmium would save many people from Alzheimer's disease. A simple switch from tap or bottled water to filtered water can significantly cut your cadmium exposure, as well as your exposure to the other harmful metals listed above.

When you're selecting a water filtration pitcher or system, be sure to obtain a third-party laboratory analysis showing whether the system removes aluminum, cadmium, lead, and mercury.

Super Health Bonus

Large amounts of heavy metals can impede many aspects of health. They can even impair enzymes—specialized proteins within your body that control almost every biochemical function. So reducing your exposure to heavy metals can help restore almost any bodily function. While it may not be possible to immediately feel the difference, many people report having fewer headaches, less "brain fog," and more energy once they've made an effort to reduce their heavy metal exposure.

60-SECOND BRAIN HEALTH TIP #7:

Skip the Antacids to Avoid Brain-Damaging Aluminum

Eliminate one of the main sources of metals that have been linked to Alzheimer's disease.

While we discussed the damaging effects of heavy metals in the previous tip, the use of antacids is so commonplace that it warrants additional discussion. Before you grab that antacid tablet to cope with indigestion, consider that most antacids contain excessively high amounts of aluminum. Aluminum is not actually a heavy metal, but it *is* a potentially brain-damaging metal. While the link between aluminum and brain diseases is still controversial, several studies note abnormally high concentrations of aluminum in people diagnosed with Alzheimer's. Some even note 30 times the level of aluminum as their healthy counterparts. As early as 45 years ago, researchers made a startling discovery: When scientists injected aluminum into the brains of rabbits used for laboratory research, the aluminum triggered the formation of neurofibrillary tangles—the same type of damage found in people with Alzheimer's disease.[22]

While there is debate about whether aluminum is a cause of the disease, research shows that it can interrupt more than 50 necessary brain chemical reactions.[23] Additionally, aluminum can cross the blood–brain barrier—a brain-protecting mechanism—to cause brain and nerve cell death. Once aluminum enters your brain, it promotes inflammation by causing the formation of brain-damaging free radicals and inducing toxic reactions. As previously mentioned, some studies indicate that the brains of Alzheimer's patients contain 30 times the level of aluminum as their healthy counterparts, so it is imperative to consider aluminum to be a possible factor in the disease.[24] Additional research links aluminum to the increasing incidence of Parkinson's disease, as well.[25]

While researchers continue to assess aluminum's connection to brain diseases, it is important to reduce your exposure to the toxic metal. One of the easiest ways to reduce your exposure is to stop using antacids. Most antacid preparations used for indigestion contain excessive amounts of aluminum.

How to Benefit

Stop using antacids. If your digestive troubles seem unbearable, choose a more natural option than aluminum-containing commercially available antacids, such as this simple, all-natural alternative: Mix 1 teaspoon of aluminum-free baking soda into ½ cup of water. Sip slowly when suffering from indigestion.

However, regularly taking antacids, even this all-natural alternative, is not healthy, as antacids interfere with proper digestion. If you consistently have indigestion, you may need to choose less complex meal combinations, eat smaller amounts of food at a single meal, avoid eating desserts or sweets directly after a meal, drink less water with meals, or take a full-spectrum digestive enzyme with meals. Keep in mind that most people observe that their digestive troubles—and indigestion in particular—greatly improve on this plan. That's because following the Principles will help you restore your body's natural healing functions.

Antacids aren't the only sources of aluminum to avoid. Stop using aluminum cookware, as well, since the aluminum can leach into the foods you cook in it. A study conducted by the University of Cincinnati Medical Center found that when tomatoes are cooked in aluminum cookware, the aluminum content per serving increases by 2 to 4 milligrams.[26] Be sure to check out 60-Second Brain Health Tip #6 on page 62 to discover aluminum's many other hiding places.

Some antacids that may contain aluminum include Aludrox, Di-Gel, Gaviscon, Gelusil, Maalox, Magalox, Mylanta, Pepto-Bismol, Remegel, and Rolaids.[27] This is not an exhaustive list; these are simply the antacids tested.

Super Health Bonus

Avoiding antacids and other sources of aluminum can often improve digestive problems. Excess aluminum in the body can be linked with gastrointestinal irritation, indigestion, and nausea, all of which may improve over time as your body eliminates the aluminum.

60-SECOND BRAIN HEALTH TIP #8:
Eliminate Chemical Scents for a Sensational Brain

You brain may be affected much more than you imagine when you spritz that perfume or cologne.

If you've walked through a department store lately, you have probably been overwhelmed by the perfume section. Whether you are obsessed with Obsession, a believer in Believe, or consumed by L'Air du Temps, the smell of perfumes and colognes can be overwhelming. The toxic effects of the fragrances in perfumes and other scented products can also be overwhelming.

More than 500 chemicals can potentially be used while listing the single word "fragrance" on a label. Fragrances are found in many products, not just perfumes and colognes: "air fresheners," room deodorizers, cosmetics, fabric softeners, laundry detergents, candles, and many other places. Manufacturers are not required to list ingredients on the labels of these products, nor do they have to reveal to regulating authorities the specific ingredients that qualify as "fragrance," because they are protected as trade secrets.

Some of the most common chemicals in perfumes are ethanol, acetaldehyde, benzaldehyde, benzyl acetate, alpha-Pinene, acetone, benzyl alcohol, ethyl acetate, linalool, alpha-Terpinene, methylene chloride, styrene oxide, dimethyl sulphate, alpha-Terpineol, camphor, and limonene. Some of these chemicals cause irritability, mental vagueness, muscle pain, asthma, bloating, joint aches, sinus pain, fatigue, sore throat, eye irritation, gastrointestinal problems, laryngitis, headaches, dizziness, swollen lymph nodes, spikes in blood pressure, coughing, and burning or itching skin irritations.

And that's just the tip of the iceberg. Acetaldehyde is a probable human carcinogen. In animal studies, it crossed the placenta to an unborn fetus. The chemical industry's own Material Safety Data Sheets list headaches, tremors, convulsions, and even death as possible effects of exposure to acetonitrile, another common fragrance ingredient. In animal studies, styrene oxide causes depression. Toluene (also known as methylbenzene) is a well-established neurotoxin that can cause loss of muscle control, brain damage, headaches, memory loss, and problems with speech, hearing, and vision—many symptoms that mimic brain diseases. And musk tetralin has been shown to actually cause brain cell and spinal cord degeneration.

Research confirms that many of the ingredients in fragrances are neurotoxins, meaning they have poisonous effects on your brain and nervous system.

Additional studies link other negative emotional, mental, and physical symptoms to various fragrance ingredients. Until recently, scientists believed that the brain was protected by the blood–brain barrier. But studies show that this system allows many environmental toxins, including those found in perfumes and other scented products, to access your delicate brain, and that once they're in your brain, these chemicals can take decades to eliminate—decades that can result in the formation of inflammation.

Some fragrance ingredients disrupt your natural brain hormonal balance, causing any number of possible emotional concerns, including anxiety, mood swings, and depression. Feeling down? It could be the scent you're wearing.

Not all scented products are created equal. Commercial brands of perfumes and colognes are primarily made from synthetic chemicals. Even many natural products contain synthetic fragrance ingredients, so it's important to start reading labels on personal care products. If there's no ingredients list, the manufacturer may have something to hide. Also, beware of "fragrance oils" masquerading as essential oils. The former are synthetic, while the latter are derived from flowers, leaves, and other natural substances. Fragrance oils are not only found in many perfumes and colognes, they are also found in air fresheners and deodorizers, laundry soaps, fabric softeners, scented candles, and other scented products.

If you're still not convinced that these commonly available products are putting your brain at risk, here are eight neurotoxins found in most fabric softeners—and eight reasons to switch to natural options.

1. **Alpha-Terpineol.** This chemical has been linked to disorders of the brain and nervous system, loss of muscle control, depression, and headaches.

2. **Benzyl acetate.** Benzyl acetate has been linked to cancer of the pancreas.

3. **Benzyl alcohol.** Benzyl alcohol is found in most common brands of fabric softeners, and it has been linked to headaches, nausea, vomiting,

dizziness, and depression, as well as disorders of the brain and nervous system.

4. **Chloroform.** Chloroform is on the Environmental Protection Agency's list of hazardous wastes because it has been identified as a carcinogen and neurotoxin (a substance toxic to the brain and nervous system).

5. **Ethanol.** Ethanol is also on the EPA's hazardous waste list because of its ability to cause brain and nervous system disorders.

6. **Ethyl acetate.** This toxic chemical causes headaches and is on the EPA's hazardous waste list.

7. **Linalool.** In studies, this chemical caused loss of muscle coordination, nervous system and brain disorders, and depression.

8. **Pentane.** Pentane is a toxic chemical that causes headaches, nausea, dizziness, fatigue, drowsiness, and depression.

The standard argument in favor of using fabric softeners is that the amount of the chemicals to which a person is exposed is insufficient to cause harm. But studies are showing that even small amounts of these toxins can have serious effects. So think twice before you add that dryer sheet or liquid fabric softener to your laundry, particularly if you have children whose developing brains are more vulnerable to the effects of toxins.

Shakespeare claimed: "That which we call a rose by any other name would smell as sweet." Thanks to today's chemical industry, that is no longer true. Worse than that, the potential brain health effects are anything but sweet.

How to Benefit

Switch your perfume to an all-natural essential oil blend. Originally, perfumes were made from essential oils, and it's only relatively recently that they've changed to be cheaper chemical varieties. Perfumes or colognes made exclusively from essential oils are not only a healthier option, but they smell better, too. And like I tell my clients, once you've had a break from the chemical versions, you'll never go back. Most people find that their sense of smell improves, and after a month or more of being chemical scent–free, they actually find the scents they once loved revolting.

So while you're selecting a natural essential oil perfume, be sure to stop using "air fresheners," "air sanitizers," and "air deodorizers." Be sure to choose unscented varieties or read the labels on products you've selected at your local health food store, since they tend to be superior to many grocery store varieties.

Choose laundry soap and natural alternatives to dryer sheets at your local health food store, as well. You can add ½ cup of baking soda to the water in your washing machine prior to adding laundry as a natural alternative to fabric softener. Not only will your brain thank you, but so will your pocketbook.

To help you avoid the worst toxic ingredients in perfumes, skin-care products, and bath and beauty products, be sure to avoid the "dirty dozen" toxic chemicals found in these products. Read labels on the products you purchase and be sure to avoid:

Artificial dyes and coal tar. These numbered dyes have names like yellow dye #5 or red dye #4 and are found in most cosmetics, body-care products, and hair dyes. Derived from coal tar, they also sometimes appear on the label as CI followed by 5 numbers, such as CI 75000. They are potentially cancer causing and contain heavy metals that are toxic to your brain.[28]

BHA and BHT. The full names of these chemicals are butylated hydroxyanisole and butylated hydroxytoluene. Both of these chemicals are suspected carcinogens and hormone disruptors.[29]

DEA, MEA, and TEA. The full names of these chemicals that make products sudsy or creamy are diethanolamine, monoethanolamine, and triethanolamine. These toxic ingredients react to form nitrosamines that are cancer causing.[30]

Dibutyl phthalate. Found in cosmetics and baby-care products, phthalates have been linked to asthma, birth defects, and cancer.[31]

Fragrance. The single ingredient "fragrance" or "parfum" can actually contain up to 500 other ingredients, many of which are petroleum by-products that have been linked to cancer, asthma, allergies, and nerve damage.[32]

Lead. Lead is rarely listed, but it's frequently found in cosmetics—especially lipsticks—so be sure yours says "lead-free." Lead is a serious threat to your brain and nervous system and is difficult to eliminate once it gets absorbed into your body.

Parabens. Used to extend the shelf lives of products, these toxins go by many names: butyl-, ethyl-, isobutyl-, methyl-, and propylparabens. The European Commission on Endocrine Disruption has identified parabens as hormone disruptors and a contributing cause of hormonally linked cancers, reproductive disorders, and other serious health issues.[33]

Petrolatum. This is found in many products, including petroleum jelly, and you guessed it: It is derived from petroleum products.

Sodium lauryl sulfate. This chemical acts as a foaming agent and is frequently found in shampoos, body washes, and soaps. It may cause cancer.[34]

Stearalkonium chloride. A common allergen found in many conditioners and creams and often cited as "natural," it is a toxic ingredient that is used because it is cheaper than natural protein ingredients.[35]

Toluene. Found in nail polish, toluene is an extremely toxic ingredient that can damage your nervous system, blood, eyes, liver, kidneys, and respiratory system. It may also affect a developing fetus.[36]

Triclosan. This chemical is added to cosmetics and body-care products as an antibacterial ingredient. I explain in my book *The Probiotic Promise* how this ingredient is contributing to the development of virulent superbugs that are resistant to our best drugs.

Super Health Bonus

Since most scented products are known endocrine disruptors, by eliminating them, you'll probably feel improvements in hormonal balance and experience better mood balance, too.

60-SECOND BRAIN HEALTH TIP #9:

Switch Fabric Softeners for Superb Mental Functions

Discover the shocking source of common brain toxins—fabric softeners—and how you can reduce your exposure.

Since I was old enough to do my own laundry, I have never used commercial fabric softeners. As a result, I'm always astounded that anyone who uses them can think they smell good. The fake smell of "Mountain Spring" or "April Fresh" is anything but fresh smelling. I live in the mountains and was born in April, and I can honestly say that neither smells like the chemical fabric softeners and dryer sheets companies are manufacturing. The last time I inhaled the scent of spring mountain air, it made me feel energized, not headachy. So before you run for the rinse cycle with fabric softener in tow or toss a dryer sheet into your laundry, you may be surprised to learn that fabric softeners contain some of the worst brain toxins to which you're exposed. Here are the eight brain-damaging toxins lurking in your fabric softener.

1. **Alpha-Terpineol.** This chemical has been linked to disorders of the brain and nervous system, loss of muscle control, depression, and headaches.

2. **Benzyl acetate.** Benzyl acetate is a known mutagen, which means that it damages our genetic material.[37] When this happens, we may become more vulnerable to disease, including brain diseases.

3. **Benzyl alcohol.** Benzyl alcohol is linked to headaches, nausea, vomiting, dizziness, and depression, as well as disorders of the brain and nervous system.

4. **Chloroform.** Chloroform is on the EPA's hazardous waste list because it has been identified as a carcinogen and neurotoxin (meaning that it is toxic to your brain and nervous system).

5. **Ethanol.** Ethanol is also on the EPA's hazardous waste list for its ability to cause brain and nervous system disorders.

6. **Ethyl acetate.** This toxin causes headaches and is on the EPA's hazardous waste list.

7. **Linalool.** In studies, this chemical caused loss of muscle coordination, nervous system and brain disorders, and depression.

8. **Pentane.** Pentane causes headaches, nausea, dizziness, fatigue, drowsiness, and depression.

How to Benefit

Skip the commercial fabric softeners and dryer sheets, as they tend to contain the above brain- and nervous system–damaging chemicals. So what are the alternatives? Most health food stores sell healthy, environmentally friendly fabric softeners. They also sell dryer balls that help reduce static and wrinkling. One-half cup of baking soda added to the washing machine and dissolved prior to adding clothes softens clothes; ½ cup of white vinegar in the wash water also works well. You can also keep clothes containing synthetic materials away from natural fabrics, since the synthetics cause static.

Super Health Bonus

If you're prone to headaches, you'll probably notice a reduction in them. Many of my clients have reported that their sense of smell seems to be heightened after they stop using fabric softeners and dryer sheets.

60-SECOND BRAIN HEALTH TIP #10:
Omit the "Air Fresheners" and Deodorizers for Better Brain Balance

Before you spritz that furniture or plug in that air "purifier," you'll want to know more about the ingredients and their effects on your brain.

Before you spray Febreze, plug in a Glade PlugIn, light a scented candle, or use some so-called air "freshening" wick, mist, aerosol, or other car or room deodorizer, think twice. You'll be shocked to learn their ingredients and the harmful brain effects they can cause.

The Natural Resources Defense Council (NRDC)—an international environmental organization—conducted a study called Clearing the Air: Hidden Hazards of Air Fresheners, in which they found that 86 percent of air fresheners tested contained dangerous phthalates.[38] Phthalates are used as plastic softeners, as antifoaming agents in aerosols, in vinyl found in children's toys, and in automobiles, paints, pesticides, cosmetics, and fragrances. Phthalates are well-established hormone disruptors that can cause reproductive abnormalities, but research also shows that they impact memory, learning, and brain health.

The Centers for Disease Control and Prevention found that the majority of the American population is routinely exposed to at least five different phthalates. Their research also shows that even if exposures to individual phthalates are small (and they may not be!), there is a significant health threat due to the combination of phthalates acting as a higher combined dose.

According to an animal study in the journal *Neuroscience*, phthalates can disrupt the normal development of the hippocampus—a part of your brain important to learning and the formation of long-term memories. Exposure to this toxic ingredient appears to reduce the number of brain cells and connections between them that form in a young animal. The brain effects may result in impaired cognitive functioning, poor memory, and significant behavioral changes throughout life.[39] While the study was conducted on animals, additional research has shown that phthalates have harmful effects on the human brain, as well.

Other human studies have linked phthalates' effects on the human brain to increased anxiety, depression, memory impairment, aggression, and behavioral changes.[40]

Phthalates are primarily added to hard plastics, including polyvinyl chloride, to make them flexible. They are found in air fresheners and deodorizers, food storage containers, children's toys, plumbing pipes, doors and windows, bottles, bank cards, and other plastic and vinyl products.

Air fresheners and deodorizers are among the worst sources of these toxic phthalates. Discover the amount of phthalates in your favorite brands of air "fresheners." Air fresheners have also been found to contain several other brain-damaging toxins, which I'll explain in further detail momentarily.

Do you feel like your brain is hitting the wal? No, that's not a typo. When I say "hitting the wal" in the context of air fresheners, I'm referring to the extremely high amounts of phthalates the NRDC found in Walgreens Air Freshener and Walgreens Scented Bouquet, along with Ozium Glycol-ized Air Sanitizer. All three of these products had more than 100 parts per million (ppm)—considered a high amount for exposure. Walgreens Scented Bouquet Air Freshener had an alarming 7,300 ppm!

But Walgreens and Ozium aren't the only culprits. Here are the amounts of phthalates found by the NRDC in some common air fresheners.

- Walgreens Scented Bouquet Air Freshener: 7,300 ppm DEP; 0.47 ppm DBP; 6.5 ppm DMP

- Walgreens Air Freshener Spray: 1,100 ppm DEP

- Ozium Glycol-ized Air Sanitizer: 360 ppm DEP; 0.15 ppm DMP

- Glade PlugIn Scented Oil Warmer: 4.5 ppm DBP

- Glade Air Infusions: 1.5 ppm DEP

- Air Wick Scented Oil: 0.75 ppm DBP; 6.3 ppm DEP; 1.6 ppm DIBP; 2.1 ppm DIHP

- Febreze NOTICEables Scented Oil: 0.19 ppm DBP; 1.5 ppm DIBP

There are many different types of phthalates, but all of the commonly used ones have been linked to health problems. The most common ones are DBP (dibutyl phthalate), DEP (diethyl phthalate), DIBP (diisobutyl phthalate), DMP (dimethyl phthalate), and DIHP (diisohexyl phthalate). As you may have noticed, air "fresheners," deodorizers, plug-ins, and scented oils all have high amounts of these toxic phthalates.

Phthalates aren't the only ingredients found in air fresheners that have damaging effects on your brain. Here are some of the ingredients found in the popular metered air fresheners—the ones that are battery-operated and pump out mists of supposed sanitizers several times an hour.[41]

Acetone. This is a common ingredient in air fresheners, as well as in nail polish remover and paint remover, and it's a serious brain and nervous system toxin.

Butane and isobutane. Yes, butane is lighter fluid, which is a serious toxin to your brain and nervous system.

Liquefied petroleum gas and petroleum distillate. It is fairly obvious why you wouldn't want to add this to your air supply. I've been half-jokingly telling my clients for years that air fresheners contain the by-products of gasoline that the oil industry can't put into vehicles. It looks like that may not be far from the truth.

Propane. Propane is a nervous system toxin known to be extremely dangerous (that's why we operate propane barbecues outdoors), yet we're spraying this stuff into our indoor air.

Perfume. This single ingredient contains up to 500 different toxic ingredients, 95 percent of which are derived from petroleum products and are linked to a whole list of serious health conditions ranging from headaches and dizziness to depression and behavioral changes.

These products frequently come with warning labels stating that deliberately inhaling the vapor of the contents "may be harmful or fatal" or that tell you to "Avoid inhaling spray mist or vapor." How are we supposed to avoid inhaling something that is constantly being forced into our air? And if inhaling the vapors may be harmful or fatal, why are we intentionally adding them to our air? Seems we've been duped into thinking that we need these products to protect us from harmful bacteria or viruses, even though there is no evidence that they actually disinfect the air at all. However, the evidence is mounting that these chemical products harm us—sometimes irreparably.

How to Benefit

Stop using "air fresheners," "air sanitizers," and "air deodorizers." Even many "natural" or "unscented" products simply use extra ingredients to mask the scents. And don't be duped by the ridiculous advertisements that show unscientific "studies" proving the so-called effectiveness of these products. They are best kept out of your home and, if you are able, out of your office, as well.

Super Health Bonus

Phthalates have been linked with abnormally developed male genitalia, poor semen quality, low testosterone levels, and other reproductive issues. An *MSN* article found that being exposed to so-called "air fresheners" as little as once a week can increase your odds of developing asthma by as much as 71 percent and can contribute to an increase in pulmonary diseases. By limiting your exposure to phthalates and other toxins found in air fresheners, you'll reduce your risk of asthma, pulmonary diseases, and reproductive disorders, too.[42]

Brain Books in Action

NAME: Donna Cervac

AGE: 54

OCCUPATION: Restaurant owner

"I feel like the cloud has lifted. I feel sharper, I need fewer reminders, and I find that I don't repeat myself because now I remember my conversations from start to finish."

How I Got Here: When Donna Cervac's doctor took her off the birth control pills she had been taking for close to 30 years, her urge to eat sugar and white flour suddenly went away; as a result, she was thrilled to say goodbye to the 15 pounds she had been trying to lose for years. Unfortunately, in the wake of her weight loss, she found herself dealing with a massive case of brain fog.

Donna was having difficulty remembering details from conversations with her family and friends, and sometimes in the middle of the afternoon, she couldn't recall what she had intended to accomplish that day or where she had left important items. "I even forgot where I parked my car!" Looking back, Donna says that just getting through the day felt like a chore.

Nighttime wasn't any easier for Donna. She would frequently fall asleep watching television. And after going to bed, she would wake up repeatedly and often had trouble falling back asleep, which set up a vicious cycle of daytime sleepiness. Stress and anxiety only compounded these problems.

Progress Report: With no family history of brain disease, Donna was eager to try the 60 Seconds to Boost Your Brain Power Health Plan to see if it could address her symptoms. Even though she had already lost weight by cutting back on many inflammation-producing foods—like dairy, sugar, and white flour—the first week of the plan was especially hard because Donna still craved many things she couldn't have. Despite a few slipups, she drew inspiration from the support of the online community and enjoyed feeling accountable to other members of the test panel who were experiencing similar problems.

By Week 2, Donna noticed that her new lifestyle habits felt like the new norm, and her foggy episodes, as well as her migraines, had begun to lessen. This was all the motivation Donna needed to continue with the plan.

Beyond: After following the 4-week plan and seeing the results, Donna decided to stick to the changes she had made. "I've learned that there are many factors that can help or hurt my memory, and by making some relatively small changes, I've seen some big results."

Donna now reports having plenty of energy throughout the day, and she feels more focused and far less foggy. While she still feels stressed and anxious from time to time, it's far less frequent than it used to be. And her family has noticed a difference, too. "My family sees that I have more energy and seem more alert in the evenings. It's wonderful to enjoy our time together."

CHAPTER 4

WEEK 2: BOOST
Eat More of These
Brain-Boosting Superfoods

This week I will introduce you to the best brain foods to eat to give your memory and brain health a serious boost. As you will soon discover, these foods are delicious, readily available, and worth the minimal effort it takes to include them in your diet. And the rewards are great. Include at least five of these foods in your daily diet and feel free to add more than that, if you would like. The more you enjoy these brain foods, the greater the brain boost you'll receive. Of course, you can eat healthy foods other than those included in this chapter. These are simply the ones to focus on. To make it easy for you to keep track of your choices, simply place a check mark next to the brain food selections that most appeal to you. Choose at least five brain superfoods and eat them throughout the plan.

In this section, you'll learn to:

Ginger offers brain protection and reduces inflammation linked to brain diseases.

22. Give Your Brain an Oil Change (page 107)

    Boosting your omega-3 consumption strengthens brain cells and ensures the healthy transmission of memories between brain cells.

23. Go Nuts to Boost Your Memory (page 109)

    Walnuts are nutritional powerhouses that protect against brain-damaging inflammation.

24. Make like Popeye for a Powerful Brain (page 110)

    High in vitamin P, spinach prevents age-related brain decline.

25. Opt for Olives to Protect Your Brain (page 112)

    Olives and olive oil give your brain an important omega-9 boost.

26. Reap Rosemary for Brain Health Rewards (page 114)

    Research shows that rosemary is valuable for the prevention and treatment of dementia.

27. Regularly Enjoy Tomatoes for a Sharper Memory (page 116)

    Lycopene found in tomatoes significantly cuts stroke risk.

28. Rev Up Your Brain with Resveratrol (page 117)

    Resveratrol, found in grapes, protects brain cells from damage while helping to prevent Alzheimer's disease.

29. Take a Coffee Break to Maximize Your Brain Power (page 119)

    Cut your Alzheimer's risk with a daily cup of java.

30. Take a Pit Stop on the Road to Brain Health (page 123)

    Apricots, peaches, cherries, and plums protect both the watery and fatty parts of your brain from damage.

31. Get Teary-Eyed to Transform Your Brain Health (page 124)

    Onions and garlic contain powerful natural substances that protect your brain against damaging plaques linked to brain diseases.

60-SECOND BRAIN HEALTH TIP #11:

Appreciate Pomegranates for a Power-Packed Brain

Enjoying pomegranates and pomegranate juice gives your brain a potent anti-oxidant boost.

One of my favorite fruits, pomegranate, offers more than just incredible taste; it is also a nutritional and healing powerhouse. And thanks to its plentiful amounts of antioxidants, pomegranate is one of the best foods to eat when it comes to boosting your brain health.

Pomegranates rate high on the USDA's ORAC scale (oxygen radical absorbance capacity)—a measure of how well free radicals are absorbed. Free radicals are charged molecules that damage cells and tissues with which they come into contact. Foods that rate high on the ORAC scale quell free radicals quickly and effectively, before they can do serious damage.

While pomegranate is one of the most recent foods to be researched for its brain health effects, there are already numerous studies demonstrating its ability to help prevent and reverse brain damage.

One study published in the *Journal of Traditional and Complementary Medicine* found that pomegranate's high level of antioxidants was beneficial in the treatment of animals with Alzheimer's disease.[1] Another study in the journal *Current Alzheimer's Research* found that pomegranate juice consumption prevented the formation of the amyloid plaques involved in Alzheimer's disease.[2]

Pomegranate also protects against traumatic brain injury, according to new research in the journal *Life Sciences*. Scientists found that pomegranate extract worked on five levels to protect the brain against injury and damage. Pomegranate extract demonstrated significant antioxidant and anti-inflammatory effects. It also prevented the destruction of brain cells and replenished the energy available to the cells for healing and normal functions. Additionally, it protected brain DNA, making pomegranate and pomegranate juice superb brain-protecting foods to include in your ongoing brain health plan.[3] The researchers found that the more pomegranate the animals consumed, the greater their protection against brain injury.

Research shows that pomegranate fights Alzheimer's disease and traumatic brain injury, but additional research shows that it protects against stroke and high blood pressure, which is a factor for stroke. New research published in the journal *Atherosclerosis* shows that pomegranate improves the body's ability to synthesize cholesterol and destroy free radicals in the vascular system.[4] And according to research published in *Plant Foods for Human Nutrition*, pomegranate may help prevent blood pressure increases associated with eating high-fat meals.[5]

How to Benefit

There are many ways to reap the benefits of eating more pomegranates or drinking more pomegranate juice. Here are some of my favorite ones.

- Eat pomegranates fresh as a snack or a dessert alternative.
- Sprinkle pomegranate seeds on a salad for a beautiful and nutritious addition.
- Drink unsweetened bottled pomegranate juice devoid of preservatives. I recommend diluting it, using 1 part water to 1 part pomegranate juice, to avoid blood sugar spikes and crashes.
- Use a splash of pomegranate juice in your favorite salad dressing recipe to jazz up a plate of greens.
- Add some pomegranate juice to your favorite smoothie to boost the amount of antioxidants in it.
- Enjoy pomegranate juice with citrus juices or carbonated water for a delicious cocktail.

But here's a safety consideration: One animal study published in the journal *Neurobiology of Aging* found that pomegranate juice consumption aggravated Parkinson's disease in animals with the condition, so it is best avoided if you have been diagnosed with Parkinson's or if Parkinson's runs in your family.[6]

Super Health Bonus

Still not convinced about the health benefits of pomegranate? In addition to protecting your brain, enjoying pomegranates on a regular basis can protect your kidneys and liver, boost your immune system, help reduce allergic responses, regulate blood sugar, fight infections, and protect against prostate, breast, and skin cancer. Here are some examples of the exciting research that shows how pomegranates will boost your overall health while building your brain health.

Kidney protection. New research published in the journal *Renal Failure* showed that an extract of pomegranate prevented kidney damage and protected the kidneys against harmful toxins.[7]

Liver protection and regeneration. More new research published in *Toxicology and Industrial Health* showed that pomegranate juice not only protects your liver, it also helps it to regenerate after it has been damaged.[8]

Increased immunity. Pomegranates and pomegranate juice are packed with immune-boosting vitamin C—an essential nutrient for a strong and healthy immune system.

Reduced allergies. Pomegranates are high in substances called polyphenols, which have been shown to reduce the biochemical processes that are linked with allergies.

Regulation of metabolic syndrome. Research published in the journal *Food & Function* showed that pomegranate helps regulate blood sugar, improves the body's sensitivity to insulin, decreases inflammation, and improves numerous other factors involved in metabolic syndrome, which is frequently implicated in obesity and is often a precursor to diabetes. Because of these effects, pomegranate may aid weight loss.[9]

Protection against infections. New research published in the journal *Food and Chemical Toxicology* found that an extract of pomegranate increased the effectiveness of a drug used against gram-negative bacteria. Many gram-negative bacteria are known for their drug resistance.[10]

DNA defense. The antioxidants and/or phytonutrients in pomegranates also appear to interact with the body's genetic material to offer protection, which may explain part of their anticancer benefits.

Prostate-cancer protection. Research conducted at the University of California, Riverside, and published in *Translational Oncology* indicated that pomegranate juice and pomegranate extracts caused cancer cell death.[11]

Breast-cancer protection. Scientists at the University of California, Riverside, also studied the effects of pomegranate juice and three of its nutritional components—luteolin, ellagic acid, and punicic acid—against breast cancer. They published their results in the journal *Breast Cancer Research and Treatment* and concluded that pomegranate juice and its extracts "are potentially a very effective treatment to prevent cancer progression."[12]

Skin-cancer protection. Consumption of pomegranate was associated with a decrease in both main types of skin cancer, basal cell carcinoma and squamous cell carcinoma, according to new research in the *British Journal of Dermatology*.[13]

60-SECOND BRAIN HEALTH TIP #12:
Eat Cherries to Power Up Your Brain Protection

Compounds in cherries protect both the watery and fatty parts of your brain from damage.

Who doesn't love cherries? They're like nature's own all-natural candy, but without the guilt. And now there's more reason than ever to enjoy cherries: They help to protect your brain from harmful toxins and even give your body a boost of antioxidants that quell inflammation and prevent brain damage.

Almost daily, scientists discover new phytochemicals (natural substances found in plants) that fight aging and disease. The best way to obtain these thousands of varied substances is to eat a variety and plentiful amount of fresh fruits and vegetables.

The USDA developed a scale of foods called the oxygen radical absorbance capacity, or ORAC, to identify superfoods that have high levels of antioxidants. Two human studies published in the *Journal of Nutrition* and the *American Journal of Nutrition* found that eating high-ORAC fruits and vegetables raises the antioxidant power of the blood by between 13 and 25 percent and may help slow the processes associated with aging of the brain and body. Cherries contain 670 ORAC units per 100 grams.

But slowing aging isn't the only health benefit cherries offer. Fruits that contain pits (see page 123 for more information on other fruits with pits) have some of the highest concentrations of flavonoids, which are protective and healing for your brain. A group of flavonoids called proanthocyanidins has demonstrated the unique capacity to protect both the fatty and nonfatty parts of your brain against damage from some environmental toxins. They appear to work by decreasing free radical activity within and between brain cells. Cherries are among the foods with the highest concentrations of these potent antioxidants.

Other research found that cherries are extremely powerful anti-inflammatories. Muraleedharan Nair, PhD, professor of natural products and chemistry at Michigan State University, found that tart cherry extract is 10 times more effective than aspirin at relieving inflammation in the body. And as you've already discovered, inflammation has been linked with many illnesses, including dementia and other brain diseases.

How to Benefit

Enjoy fresh cherries instead of your usual dessert. Pit them and add them to smoothies, salads, and even meat dishes. They add a delightful flavor to balsamic vinegar. Of course cherry pie is an option, but most cherry pies contain trans fats in their less-than-healthy crusts, as well as excessive amounts of sugar. You can also enjoy fresh or bottled cherry juice, but make sure that if you choose the latter, it isn't primarily made up of sugar or diluted with apple juice, as so many bottled juices are. You can also take 2 tablespoons daily of concentrated cherry juice, which is available in most health food stores.

Super Health Bonus

Research shows that cherries are such powerful anti-inflammatories that they even help reduce joint pain and arthritis symptoms. So if you're suffering from either of these conditions, you'll likely experience an improvement while enjoying these delicious fruits.

60-SECOND BRAIN HEALTH TIP #13:
Become a Wise Sage for a Savvy Brain

Regular consumption of sage results in a significant memory boost.

When it comes to brain health and mental acuity, you probably don't give herbs much consideration, yet they are among the most powerful brain boosters you can use. They show tremendous promise in the prevention of brain diseases and in maintaining great brain health.

More than just a seasoning for stuffing turkey, recent research shows that sage is great brain food. A British research team conducted a study of sage's therapeutic properties on a group of 44 adults between the ages of 18 and 37. Some participants were given capsules of sage oil, while others were given a placebo of sunflower oil. Results showed that those who took the sage oil performed significantly better on memory tests than those who took the placebo. The people who were given sage as part of the study showed improvements in both immediate and delayed word recall scores, as well as mood improvements. Additional research by the same scientific team led them to conclude that sage may also be helpful for those suffering from Alzheimer's disease.

How to Benefit

Fresh sage is an excellent addition to soups, stews, and chicken dishes. Sautéed in a little olive oil, it is a great accompaniment to pasta dishes, as well. I particularly like sautéed sage with butternut squash ravioli. You can also enjoy a brain-boosting whole grain "stuffing" more often than just at Thanksgiving. I add fresh, chopped sage; onions; celery; and green peppers to my favorite gluten-free whole grain mix, along with a pinch of salt, to enjoy a Thanksgiving-inspired whole grain dish year round.

Super Health Bonus

Sage has a proven history of balancing menopausal and PMS symptoms, but perhaps the most exciting benefit of sage essential oil is that it may actually protect genetic material from damage.

According to a study published in the *Journal of Agricultural and Food Chemistry*, scientists found that compounds in sage may protect cellular DNA from damage and may even stimulate DNA repair in already damaged cells. While the research is new and has not been tested on humans, this exciting advancement could help in the prevention and treatment of genetic diseases, as well as diseases with a genetic component, including cancer, heart disease, and others.

60-SECOND BRAIN HEALTH TIP #14:
Eat Blueberries for a Brilliant Brain

Regularly eating blueberries dramatically cuts inflammation and boosts memory.

When it comes to "brain food," grapes get all the attention. And while grapes are powerful brain protectors, I think it's time for blueberries to share in the acclaim. These delicious berries are brain-healing powerhouses that work to protect your brain from disease in several different ways. And increasing amounts of research show that blueberries can prevent or reverse age-related memory loss. Let's explore the ways in which blueberries work.

First, blueberries contain a group of plant nutrients called flavonoids, which protect both the watery and the fatty parts of your brain against free radical damage. You may recall that your brain is about 60 percent fat, so it's equally important to protect both parts. Typically, fat-soluble vitamins tend to protect the fatty part of your brain, so it's uncommon to find a food that is low in fat yet protects your brain so well. Blueberries are among the foods with the highest concentrations of the flavonoids called proanthocyanidins. Proanthocyanidins give blueberries their rich blue color and act as antioxidants that destroy free radicals linked to aging and disease.

Proanthocyanidins are likely the compounds responsible for the impressive brain health results blueberries demonstrated in many studies. Whatever the mechanism at work, it's clear from animal studies that those given an extract of blueberries had less motor skill decline and performed better on memory tests than animals not given the blueberries. Researchers concluded that compounds in blueberries may reverse some age-related memory loss and motor skill decline.

Second, blueberries contain salicylic acid—the natural version of aspirin—which helps prevent arterial clogging linked to stroke. It also acts as an anti-inflammatory to take down inflammation, which is an underlying factor in many brain diseases.

Third, other as-yet-unidentified compounds in blueberries help to increase levels of heat shock proteins in your body. Heat shock proteins (or stress proteins, as they are also called) are used by your body to address sudden internal temperature increases and other stresses. They also play a role in assembling and transporting proteins within your body and protecting cells. Heat shock proteins tend to decrease as we age. When levels become too low, the result is cellular inflammation and damage, including damage to your brain. Research shows that blueberries help to restore heat shock proteins and that if you eat blueberries regularly, inflammation tends to lessen.[14]

There is a fourth mechanism by which blueberries improve brain health: Consuming blueberries on a regular basis increases your body's production of the feel-good brain chemical messenger called dopamine. Dopamine helps to control your brain's reward and pleasure center, and levels tend to be low in people with brain diseases such as Parkinson's.

Finally, blueberries are packed with the brain-boosting and protecting vitamin E, niacin, and folate, and they contain the minerals magnesium, manganese, and potassium. Check out 60-Second Brain Health Tips #47 (page 172), #45 (page 165), #50 (page 178), #19 (page 101), and #11 (page 84) for more information on each of these nutrients .

How to Benefit

Eat at least ½ cup of blueberries daily, at least 5 days a week. They can be fresh or frozen but should not be canned or sweetened. It's easy to add blueberries to smoothies or to blend them and make ice pops in freezer molds. One of my favorite ways to enjoy blueberries is to slightly thaw frozen ones and snack on them as a delicious sorbet-like dessert. You can also blend them into a pudding, add them to your breakfast cereal, enjoy them atop a salad, or just snack on them on their own. They taste amazing while protecting your brain.

Super Health Bonus

In addition to their many other nutrients, blueberries are a rich source of ellagic acid, a phytonutrient that has proven anticancer and genetic material protection capabilities. It also encourages a healthy rate of apoptosis—the method by which your body seeks out and destroys harmful or damaged cells, such as cancer cells. This process helps reduce cancer risk.

60-SECOND BRAIN HEALTH TIP #15:
Chomp on Celery to Prevent Memory Lapses

Containing 20 anti-inflammatory compounds, celery and celery seeds are brain-boosting superstars.

Celery might just be the most overlooked brain health superfood. Perhaps it is because affordable, readily available celery is just too commonplace to even be considered. But when it comes to your brain, you'll want to give celery a second thought. It is definitely a brain superfood.

Over 900 years ago, Hildegard von Bingen, a writer, scientist, musician, and nun, wrote about celery's anti-inflammatory properties. But it was only much more recently that scientists have proven what she knew almost a millennium ago. James Duke, PhD, author of *The Green Pharmacy* and world-renowned botanist, discovered that both celery and celery seeds contain more than 20 natural anti-inflammatory compounds, including an extremely potent one known as apigenin. These anti-inflammatories help reduce brain inflammation that can occur as you age and make you more vulnerable to memory lapses and brain decline.

How to Benefit

Celery is one of the most versatile foods, making it simple to add to your daily diet. You can juice celery in a juicer or blender. (If you're using a blender, you'll want to add a bit of water and drink it immediately, as the fiber quickly bulks up.) Add chopped celery or celery seeds to soups or stews. My sister blends pieces of celery into her excellent Caesar salad dressing to thicken it and give it a hint of celery taste, along with all of the health benefits. You can also enjoy raw celery crudités with almond butter, hummus, or your favorite dip or spread, or add chopped, raw celery to salads.

Use either celery seeds or celery as a salt substitute in recipes to obtain the anti-inflammatory benefits. Both the seeds and the stalks have a naturally salty flavor that lends itself to many dishes. One of my favorite appetizers to have in place of garlic bread is celery bread. It's made the same as garlic bread but uses celery seeds in place of the garlic. Simply brush olive oil on whole grain gluten-free bread, sprinkle with celery seeds, and bake until golden.

Super Health Bonus

You can also reap the benefits of celery seeds in supplement form. Some supplement formulations for the arthritic condition gout, which is primarily experienced as pain in your big toe, contain this valuable anti-inflammatory remedy. That's because celery and celery seeds are proven arthritis remedies.

60-SECOND BRAIN HEALTH TIP #16:

Consider the Curry Factor for a Brain Boost

Curcumin found in curry provides potent protection against brain diseases.

Taste isn't the only reason to enjoy your favorite Indian curry dishes: They typically contain the yellow-colored spice known as turmeric—a powerful food that helps protect your brain from disease.

Research conducted by Greg Cole, PhD, associate director of the Mary S. Easton Center for Alzheimer's Disease Research at UCLA, showed that curcumin, the pigment that gives turmeric its signature yellow color, is also a potent weapon against inflammation and plaque buildup in the brain.[15] Inflammation and plaque have been linked to serious brain diseases, including Alzheimer's. Early evidence of the link between inflammation and Alzheimer's disease began when University of British Columbia researcher Patrick McGeer and Sun Health Research Institute, Arizona, researcher Jo Rogers explored a decade of hospital drug records and found that arthritis patients who were regularly treated with strong anti-inflammatory drugs were seven times less likely to develop Alzheimer's.[16]

But strong arthritis drugs aren't a great option, as they are linked with serious side effects. Some of the drugs in this class of medications, known as COX-2 inhibitors, were temporarily pulled from the market due to the number of deaths associated with them. Fortunately, turmeric is both a COX-2 inhibitor and works on an additional level of inflammation. Prostaglandins, the chemical messengers that are frequently responsible for inflammation in your body, are made by two enzymes known as cyclooxygenase-1 (COX-1) and cyclooxygenase-2 (COX-2). While the arthritis drugs work on the COX-2 enzymes, turmeric works on both enzymes to stop inflammation in its tracks. Even better, turmeric doesn't have the negative side effects of the drugs.

Additionally, research conducted by a medical team at a graduate school at Kanazawa University, Japan, demonstrated that curcumin prevents the development of a substance called beta amyloid in the brain. This substance is considered to be a causative factor for Alzheimer's disease.[17]

Additional studies are reaching similar positive results. In an animal study published in the *Journal of Neuroscience Research*, scientists found that curcumin improved spatial learning and memory.[18]

In another study, three Alzheimer's patients with severe symptoms that included dementia, irritability, agitation, anxiety, and apathy were given turmeric supplements. After taking 764 milligrams (mg) of turmeric with 100 mg per day of curcumin for 12 weeks, they "started recovering from these symptoms without any adverse reaction in the clinical symptom and laboratory data." After 3 months of treatment, the patients' symptoms and their reliance on caregivers significantly decreased. After 1 year of treatment, two of the patients recognized their family members, though they were unable to do so at the outset of the study. In one of the cases, the person had a 17 percent improvement on their mini-mental state examination (MMSE) score.[19] The MMSE is a 30-point questionnaire that is used extensively in clinical studies and research to measure cognitive impairment.

How to Benefit

The easiest way to enjoy the benefits of curcumin is to add turmeric to your favorite curry soup or stew. For best results treating or preventing brain diseases, you may need more of the active ingredient than is typically present in most foods. In that case, take a standardized extract with at least 1,200 mg of curcumin content per day. There are currently no known undesirable effects, even with large doses. Most of my clients report tremendous memory improvements simply by taking curcumin supplements and eating more turmeric as part of their daily diets.

Super Health Bonus

One of turmeric's many properties is its ability to suppress pain through the same mechanism as the pain-killing COX-1 and COX-2 inhibitor drugs primarily used for pain. Turmeric also has powerful anti-inflammatory properties. Recent research indicates that ingesting 1,200 mg of curcumin, the main therapeutic constituent of the spice turmeric, had the same effect as taking 300 mg of the potent anti-inflammatory drug phenylbutazone.[20] Unlike phenylbutazone, which is highly toxic and has been removed from the marketplace, turmeric is safe for use.

Turmeric's potent pain-fighting and anti-inflammatory properties work throughout your body, without the worry of the harmful side effects linked to drugs. Because research also shows that turmeric depletes nerve endings of substance P, a pain neurotransmitter, thereby reducing pain, you are likely to experience less pain and inflammation throughout your body while taking this supplement and/or using turmeric in your cooking.

60-SECOND BRAIN HEALTH TIP #17:
Drink Tea for Two Hemispheres

Catechins found in tea prevent damage to and destruction of brain cells.

Perhaps the Queen of England's afternoon tea break has helped to keep her mind sharp as she has aged? Black, green, and white tea all have significant amounts of anti-inflammatory and antioxidant compounds called catechins, which makes them a great choice for a healthy brain. These natural phyto-chemicals have shown great promise as brain protectors in recent studies.[21]

In other research, scientists found that people who drank two or more cups of tea each day were less likely to develop Parkinson's disease.[22] Green tea extract reduced neuron loss in the area of the brain that is damaged in Parkinson's disease.[23]

Still further research found that green tea contains potent antioxidants that fight free radicals with 20 times the power of vitamin E. Free radicals react with healthy cells in the brain, causing damage, so lessening their num-bers helps reduce damage to brain cells. Green tea also lowers the risk of blood clots and clumping linked to stroke. But it's not just its antioxidant effects that help reduce your risk of stroke. Green tea also prevents cholesterol buildup in arteries and helps prevent cardiovascular disease. According to research in the *Journal of Biological Chemistry*, EGCG (epigallocatechin gallate, a special type of plant nutrient found in black, green, and white tea) helps prevent fat buildup in arteries.[24] If you've heard about the many health benefits of green tea, these benefits are primarily due to its EGCG. White and black tea also contain this substance; however, black tea typically contains less than white or green tea.

Another study suggests that regular caffeine exposure may counteract the age-related degenerative process in the brain that leads to a loss of the brain chemical dopamine, a key factor in Parkinson's.[25]

There's still more great news about tea-drinking's ability to improve your brain health: EGCG improves insulin use in your body to prevent blood sugar spikes and crashes that can result in fatigue, irritability, and cravings for unhealthy foods. And you may recall from our earlier discussions that stable blood sugar levels are imperative to ensure that your brain has a steady flow of energy that lets it function properly. Stable blood sugar also reduces the likelihood that inflammation will form in your brain.

How to Benefit

Add 1 or 2 teaspoons of green tea leaves to a cup of boiled water, preferably in a tea strainer. Let steep for 5 minutes. Pour over ice, if you prefer a cold beverage. Most experts recommend 3 cups daily. And don't worry: Green tea contains a lot less caffeine than coffee or black tea.

If you're not wild about the flavor, try a few different kinds. Try it iced or hot. Add some of the natural herb stevia to sweeten it, if you want a sweeter drink. I wasn't crazy about green tea the first few times I tried it, but now I love it over ice with a squeeze of fresh lemon and a few drops of stevia. Voilà—green tea lemonade! Mmmmm. Even green tea haters love this drink.

Super Health Bonus

Because tea (especially green and white tea) contains potent antioxidants that kill free radicals, drinking it may help reduce the incidence of many serious chronic illnesses, including arthritis, diabetes, and cancer.

60-SECOND BRAIN HEALTH TIP #18:
Eat More Fiber for Fabulous Mental Functions

Fiber works in four different ways to boost brain health.

Okay, I know you're probably wondering how fiber boosts your mental functions. After all, doesn't fiber just work on the bowels? While fiber certainly helps keep your bowels regular, it is also critical to the health of your brain in multiple ways.

First, it helps prevent the backup of waste materials in your intestines, which would otherwise lead to toxins moving through your intestinal walls and into your blood, and ultimately to your brain. That's because the intestinal walls are where nutrients are absorbed into your bloodstream. If your gut walls are compacted with waste matter, this toxic waste is absorbed instead. Fiber helps to eliminate these toxic waste materials before they can do damage.

Second, fiber also helps your intestines eliminate bacterial or yeast overgrowth, the by-products of which can transfer into your blood. Fiber helps to push these harmful infections out of your body.

Third, fiber binds to specific toxins in your body to escort them out. Different types of fiber bind to different toxins. For example, rice bran and spinach fiber bind to toxic polychlorinated biphenyls; pectin from apples and oranges, as well as carrot and cabbage fibers, bind to the heavy metal lead. These fibers help eliminate these toxins from your body so they are less capable of accessing your brain.[26]

Fourth, fiber also helps to regulate the release of glucose by preventing rapid blood sugar spikes. This helps to ensure that your brain has a steady supply of energy, rather than the energy surges and crashes common to people consuming the Standard American Diet.

How to Benefit

Legumes are some of the greatest sources of fiber. It is easy to add chickpeas, lentils, kidney beans, navy beans, or other beans to your diet to reap the nutritional benefits they offer. Whole grains are also excellent sources of fiber. Most fruits and vegetables contain beneficial amounts of fiber, giving you one more reason to consume them.

To help you get enough fiber, I've compiled a list of my top whole food, gluten-free sources of fiber. Most other lists include different types of bran, but bran is still fairly processed, and I always prefer whole food options over processed foods. Here are my preferred readily available, gluten-free, fiber-rich whole foods.

Beans, Beans the Magical Fruit. Few foods can compare with beans when it comes to fiber. If you're not already striving to get a cup of beans into your daily diet, now might be a good time to start. Here are the fiber grams per cup of some good choices:

Adzuki beans	17 g	Lentils	16 g
Black beans	15 g	Navy beans	19 g
Garbanzo beans (chickpeas)	12 g	Pinto beans	15 g
Kidney beans	16 g		

Go Nuts for Nuts. Nuts are an excellent fiber-rich whole food, provided you eat the raw, unsalted ones found in the refrigerator section of your natural food store. Because they contain volatile oils, most nuts sold elsewhere have been overheated during processing or exposed to excessive amounts of heat during storage. The result: rancid oils. I haven't included peanuts because they are especially vulnerable to aflatoxins—a type of mold that is damaging to the body. Here are the fiber grams per 1-ounce serving of my preferred picks:

Almonds	4 g	Pine nuts	12 g
Brazil nuts	12 g	Pistachios	3 g
Cashews	1 g	Walnuts	2 g

The Seed-y Side of Healthy Eating. Most people rarely give seeds a second thought, yet they are powerhouses of healthy fats, protein, and, of course, fiber. Since seeds tend to be used in different ways and in different quantities, I've listed the serving sizes for some of the best seeds and the fiber grams per serving.

Chia seeds (2 tablespoons)	10 g	Pumpkin seeds (½ cup)	3 g
Flaxseeds (2 tablespoons)	4 g	Sesame seeds (¼ cup)	4 g
Hemp seeds (2 tablespoons)	2 g	Sunflower seeds (½ cup)	6 g

Beautiful Berries. Not only do berries taste great, but they are high in fiber, too. Here are the fiber grams per 1-cup serving of some of the best berries to choose to maximize your fiber intake.

Blackberries	8 g	Raspberries	8 g
Blueberries	4 g	Strawberries	3 g
Elderberries	10 g		

The Whole Grain and Nothing But. Because many people suffer from gluten sensitivities, I've listed the top whole, gluten-free, high-fiber grains and their fiber grams per 1-cup cooked serving.

Amaranth	5 g	Millet	2 g
Brown rice	4 g	Oats	8 g
Buckwheat groats	5 g	Quinoa	5 g

Leafy Greens and Squash. Some of the best vegetable sources of fiber include leafy greens and squashes. Here are their fiber grams per 1-cup cooked serving:

Collard greens	5 g	Butternut squash	6 g
Kale	3 g	Hubbard squash	7 g
Spinach	5 g	Spaghetti squash	2 g
Swiss chard	4 g	Summer squash	5 g
Acorn squash	9 g	Zucchini	3 g

Super Health Bonus

Your bowels will love you for adding more fiber to your diet. And the additional fiber also means you'll significantly decrease your risk of bowel disorders, including colon cancer.

60-SECOND BRAIN HEALTH TIP #19:
Eat More Beans to Boost Cognition

Beans are high in critical nutrients that eliminate brain-damaging toxic compounds.

Beans could just be the most underrated food in your diet. Most types of beans have high levels of vitamin B_6 and folate, both of which help to lessen levels of homocysteine in your body. High homocysteine levels often indicate an increased risk of heart disease, stroke, and accelerated aging. The beans that are highest in vitamin B_6 and folate are kidney beans and black beans.

Beans are usually high in the B vitamin thiamin, which is integral to energy production and brain cell and cognitive function. Also known as vitamin B_1, thiamin is needed to make an important brain messenger substance called acetylcholine, making this vitamin imperative to healthy memory function.[27]

Kidney beans are high in the mineral manganese, which your body needs to make an important enzyme called superoxide dismutase, or SOD, as it is sometimes known. SOD disarms free radicals produced in the energy centers of your cells, thereby improving energy production and lessening oxidative damage in your body. A cup of kidney beans supplies you with almost one-quarter of the recommended daily dose of manganese.

A large-scale study called the Normative Aging Study linked high dietary folate in foods like beans with less cognitive decline.[28]

How to Benefit

It's easy to get at least ½ cup of beans in your diet every day. Add cooked chickpeas to a salad, enjoy hummus with vegetable crudités, or puree chickpeas with roasted red peppers and a bit of sea salt to enjoy in place of mashed potatoes. Add a handful of beans or lentils to your favorite soups, stews, casseroles, curries, tacos, fajitas, and wraps. And of course, there's always the old standby: chili. Navy beans have the highest amount of fiber at 19 grams per cup, and kidney beans have 16 grams, but all beans are rich in fiber, so any beans will do. Use lentils or chickpeas to make veggie burgers, or use chickpea flour in baked goods.

Super Health Bonus

Beans' blood sugar–regulating effects will have the added bonus of keeping your energy balanced throughout the day. And new research in the *European Journal of Nutrition* shows that eating a diet high in legumes such as lentils and chickpeas can help your body burn excess body fat. That's because beans contain protein and fiber, both of which help stabilize blood sugar levels. Avoiding blood sugar spikes and drops ensures that your body stops storing extra pounds, particularly around your waistline. Beans may help restore a healthy weight in another way, as well. In one study, participants reported greater dietary satisfaction and ate fewer processed foods when chickpeas (also known as garbanzo beans) were included in their diets.

60-SECOND BRAIN HEALTH TIP #20:

Enjoy an Apple a Day to Keep Dementia at Bay

A daily apple or serving of apple juice halts brain decline by boosting essential brain hormones.

We've all heard the old adage "an apple a day keeps the doctor away," and provided that the apple is an organic one, it may actually be true, when it comes to brain health.

Research published in the *American Journal of Alzheimer's Disease & Other Dementias* found that people with moderate to severe Alzheimer's who drank two 4-ounce cups of apple juice daily had a 27 percent reduction in agitation, anxiety, and delusion.[29] A study in the *Journal of Nutrition, Health & Aging* found that regular apple juice consumption compensated for the dietary and genetic deficiencies that promote brain degeneration.[30]

Another study published in the *Journal of Alzheimer's Disease* found that supplementing animals' diets with apple juice concentrate prevented the free radical damage and cognitive decline common in Alzheimer's disease. It also helped the animals to maintain healthy acetylcholine levels, while animals whose diets were not supplemented with the apple juice had a significant decline in the hormone.[31] Acetylcholine is your most prevalent neurotransmitter—a substance that helps brain and nerve cells communicate. Acetylcholine is involved with attention, arousal, and muscle activation.[32]

While apples and apple juice work directly on reducing free radical damage and maintaining optimal brain levels of acetylcholine, they also work to maintain a powerful brain by keeping cholesterol levels healthy and preventing stroke. Scientists at BHF Health Promotion Research Group, Nuffield Department of Population Health, at the University of Oxford, in England, compared the effects of eating one daily apple to taking statin drugs (used to lower cholesterol levels) among adults age 50 and up.

The study participants made no other dietary or lifestyle changes, and their mortality rates from strokes and heart attacks were recorded. The results of the study were published in the *BMJ*. Scientists found that eating an apple a day or taking statin drugs daily resulted in an equivalent reduction in mortality. The scientists also estimate that if 70 percent of the over-50 population of the United Kingdom simply ate one apple daily, 8,500 deaths every year due to heart attack or stroke would be averted. And if 90 percent of the British population over age 50 ate a daily apple, the number of lives saved would climb to 11,000 annually. Similar results could be expected in North America.

The great news is that if people ate a daily apple instead of taking statin drugs to prevent strokes and heart attacks, there would not be an increase in any of the serious health conditions linked to statin drug use. The researchers concluded, "An apple a day or a statin a day is equally likely to keep the doctor away." They added, "We find that a 150-year-old proverb is able to match modern medicine and is likely to have fewer side effects."[33]

Not only are apples and apple juice able to help boost brain health, new research also shows that the addition of apple cider vinegar to your diet will help lower high cholesterol levels that can increase stroke risk. In a study published in the *Journal of Membrane Biology*, researchers studied the effects of a high-cholesterol diet on animals fed apple cider vinegar versus animals that only ate the high-cholesterol diet. They found that the apple cider vinegar exerted a protective effect against the high-cholesterol diet.[34]

How to Benefit

Apples truly are nature's fast food. They come ready to eat in a package that is easy to take almost anywhere. They simply need a quick wash. So it is easy to reap their many health benefits, including giving your brain a boost and providing the protection it needs against brain diseases. Add an apple to your lunch, have one as a snack on a break from work, or eat one as an evening treat to quell a sweet tooth. Use applesauce in your baking to reduce the amount of sugar needed. (This will take some adjustment of dry and wet ingredients.) You can also blend apple cider vinegar with a little olive oil, sea salt, and some herbs to make a delicious and nutritious salad dressing.

Super Health Bonus

An apple a day can significantly cut your risk of heart disease. Apples, apple juice, and apple cider vinegar contain the nutrient chlorogenic acid. According to the journal *Biochemical Pharmacology*, chlorogenic acid helps prevent LDL cholesterol, also known as the "bad cholesterol," from oxidizing, and oxidation is an important step in the progression of heart disease.[35] And adding apple cider vinegar to your daily diet has been shown in research to help you lose weight. According to research in the *European Journal of Clinical Nutrition*, apple cider vinegar can help reduce the number of calories eaten at a meal by between 200 and 275.[36] Additional study results published in the journal *Bioscience, Biotechnology, and Biochemistry* also showed that apple cider vinegar helped with weight loss in obese individuals.[37]

60-SECOND BRAIN HEALTH TIP #21:
Enjoy Ginger to Take Down Inflammation

Ginger offers brain protection and reduces inflammation linked to brain diseases.

Not just great in stir-fries, ginger is one herb that can do more than add flavor and spice to just about any dish; it also exhibits antioxidant effects and the ability to lessen the formation of inflammation in the brain. Ginger contains gingerols—potent anti-inflammatory compounds that are responsible for the herb's magic. A study in the journal *Life Sciences* found that ginger offers protection against free radicals, which have the potential to be a serious threat to brain health.

A study conducted by Dr. Honlei Chen and his colleagues at the Harvard T. H. Chan School of Public Health suggests that inflammation plays an important role in the development of Parkinson's disease.[38] Inflammatory processes also appear in the development of Alzheimer's disease. Therefore, foods that contain anti-inflammatory compounds play an important role in the prevention of brain diseases and maintenance of a healthy brain.

According to Dr. Krishna C. Srivastava of the University of Southern Denmark, ginger is superior to nonsteroidal anti-inflammatory drugs (NSAIDs) in alleviating inflammation. NSAIDs work on one level, blocking the substances that cause inflammation, while ginger works on at least two mechanisms: (1) ginger blocks the formation of inflammatory compounds, and (2) ginger has antioxidant properties that actually break down inflammation and acidity in the body.[39] This is promising research because anti-inflammatory drugs are being considered for use with inflammation-related brain diseases.

Research also shows that ginger reduces harmful cholesterol in your blood, thereby reducing your risk of stroke. Researchers studied 95 people with high triglycerides, high LDL cholesterol (known as the "bad cholesterol"), and low HDL cholesterol (known as the "good cholesterol"). They divided the participants into two groups: The first group took 1,000 milligrams of ginger three times a day; the other group took a placebo. After 45 days, participants taking the ginger had a greater drop in LDL cholesterol and a greater increase in HDL cholesterol than the group taking the placebo.[40]

How to Benefit

The easiest way to enjoy the benefits of ginger is to grate 2 tablespoons of fresh ginger and add it to a cup of boiling water. Steep and strain. Enjoy a cup of this warming ginger tea with a touch of honey or a few drops of stevia. You can also add freshly grated ginger to soups, stir-fries, vegetables, and other dishes to pack extra brain health into your meals. Additionally, you can purchase ginger supplements to help you obtain a higher dosage of this excellent anti-inflammatory herb. Follow package instructions.

Super Health Bonus

If you're suffering from joint or muscle pain, you will likely experience a reduction in pain because the gingerols in ginger are also powerful pain-relieving and anti-inflammatory compounds.

60-SECOND BRAIN HEALTH TIP #22:
Give Your Brain an Oil Change

Boosting your omega-3 consumption strengthens brain cells and ensures the healthy transmission of memories between brain cells.

Humans really are fatheads, and I don't mean that in a nasty way: About 60 percent of the human brain is fat. To maintain proper brain health, you need to get adequate fat from your diet. But not just any fat will do. Some fats damage your brain. The Standard American Diet, high in trans and hydrogenated fats, worsens inflammation in your body, and this inflammation can damage delicate brain tissues. These unhealthy fats are found in fried foods, shortening, lard, margarine, baked goods, and processed and prepared foods. But trans fats and hydrogenated fats are not the only problems.

Healthy fats help keep the lining of brain cells flexible so that memories and other brain messages can pass easily between cells. Both omega-6 and omega-3 fats are important to brain health and should be eaten in a 1-to-2 to a 2-to-1 ratio to each other. However, the average North American eats these foods in a 20-to-1 to a 40-to-1 ratio, causing a huge imbalance and resulting in an omega-3 deficiency. At this ratio, omega-6 fats can cause or worsen inflammation, leaving you with insufficient omega-3 fats to keep that inflammation under control. The typical diet, if it contains any healthy essential fatty acids, usually includes fats found in meats and poultry, or occasionally from nuts and seeds. Most of these fats are omega-6 fatty acids.

Omega-6 fatty acids are found in the highest concentrations in corn, sunflower, and safflower oils. But you are more than what you eat. I read somewhere that "you are what you eat eats." So that means if you eat a diet containing meat or poultry that was fed corn or other grains high in omega-6s, you're getting lots of omega-6s indirectly.

The best sources of omega-3 fatty acids include flaxseeds and flaxseed oil, walnuts and walnut oil, some types of algae, krill oil, and fatty cold-water fish, particularly wild salmon. Docosahexaenoic acid, a type of omega-3 fatty acid, makes up a large part of the lining of brain cells, helps to keep the cellular lining flexible enough to allow memory messages to pass between cells, promotes nerve transmission throughout your central nervous system, and protects the energy centers of your cells (called mitochondria) from damage.

Fish that contain high levels of this omega-3 fatty acid include mackerel, sardines, albacore tuna, salmon, lake trout, and herring. But be aware: Some of these fish have become contaminated with mercury and, as you learned in Chapter 2, some research links mercury to the development of brain disease. So it is important to avoid fish that consistently show up high on the mercury radar, including predatory fish like swordfish and shark, as well as sea bass, northern pike, tuna, walleye, and largemouth bass. Farmed salmon also frequently shows up with high levels of mercury, not to mention that farmed salmon often contains antibiotic residues and lower levels of the important omega-3 fatty acids.

How to Benefit

Avoid all trans fats, margarine, fried foods, and processed and prepared foods, because these are among the worst sources of brain-damaging fats. Instead, try to get a daily dose of omega-3 fatty acids from flaxseeds, flaxseed oil, chia seeds, hemp seeds, raw walnuts, mackerel, sardines, albacore tuna, salmon, lake trout, or herring. If you opt for the vegetarian options, be sure to get at least 2 teaspoons of flaxseed oil or 2 tablespoons of freshly ground flaxseeds, chia seeds, or hemp seeds daily. Also, a handful of walnuts makes a great omega-3–rich snack. If you choose to eat the fatty fish, try to eat a minimum of 4 ounces twice a week.

Super Health Bonus

Hydrogenated and trans fats aggravate inflammation in your body. Simply eliminating foods that contain these fats will help to quell inflammation elsewhere, too, including your joints. And by replacing these fats with beneficial omega-3 fatty acids, you're giving your body an anti-inflammatory boost. If you suffer from pain, you'll probably notice an improvement.

60-SECOND BRAIN HEALTH TIP #23:
Go Nuts to Boost Your Memory

Walnuts are nutritional powerhouses that protect against brain-damaging inflammation.

For better brain health, it's time to go nuts—walnuts, that is. Walnuts offer numerous brain health benefits. To start, they are packed with omega-3 fatty acids that help protect the fatty portion of your brain and quell brain inflammation, too.

Research in the *Journal of Nutrition* found that walnuts also contain natural polyphenolic compounds that act as antioxidants to destroy free radicals that could otherwise have a damaging effect on the brain. These same polyphenolic compounds reduce brain inflammation, improve signals between brain cells, and increase the generation of brain and nerve cells. As if that wasn't enough reason to start snacking on walnuts, research also shows that these compounds in walnuts have the ability to contain toxic substances so they are less likely to damage the brain.[41]

Walnuts are such powerful brain protectors that new research published in the *Journal of Alzheimer's Disease* found that eating only 1 to 1½ ounces of walnuts daily improves memory and learning, while also decreasing anxiety. The researchers indicated that the nuts are a possible preventive remedy against Alzheimer's disease.[42]

How to Benefit

Eating walnuts in your banana bread or brownies simply isn't the best way to benefit from their brain-protective properties. And it would be best to skip the little packets of walnuts found in the baking section of your grocery store. Most of these nuts have been processed at high temperatures or have been sitting around for excessive amounts of time. When the oils in walnuts go rancid or are heated to high temperatures, as they often are during processing and packaging, they taste bitter. When I tell my clients to eat more walnuts, most of them tell me they can't stand them. But time and again, when I've asked them to eat only raw, unsalted walnuts found in the refrigerator section of their health food store, they report that they *love* them. In this natural state, walnuts have a buttery, rich flavor that is as delicious as the nuts are nutritious. You can snack on a handful daily, top your favorite salads with them, or add them after you've finished cooking your favorite stir-fry.

Super Health Bonus

In addition to all of the brain health benefits of eating more walnuts, you'll reap heart rewards from enjoying these amazing nuts. That's because walnuts also quell the inflammation linked to heart disease.

60-SECOND BRAIN HEALTH TIP #24:
Make like Popeye for a Powerful Brain

High in vitamin P, spinach prevents age-related brain decline.

Do you remember episodes of the popular cartoon *Popeye*? I do. And the main thing I remember is how spinach powered up this character's muscles. The show's writers obviously knew that spinach was a serious nutritional superpower. Today's research shows that spinach doesn't just boost muscle function, it also powers up brain health.

Plant foods contain more than 4,000 naturally occurring substances called flavonoids (or vitamin P), all of which have tremendous medicinal properties. (Learn more about the brain-boosting properties of flavonoids in 60-Second Brain Health Tips #12 and #30 on pages 87 and 123, which discuss cherries and pitted fruits.) One specific group of flavonoids, polyphenols, is found in colorful fruits and vegetables, and they're present in particularly high amounts in spinach.

Polyphenols prevent oxidative damage in your brain. That means they prevent free radicals from damaging brain cells and the spaces between them. A study of rats fed extracts of blueberries, strawberries, and spinach for 8 weeks showed that these potent polyphenol-rich foods reversed some effects of age-related brain decline.[43] Other research shows that flavonoids also work with vitamin C to prevent the vitamin from breaking down in your body, allowing it to continue working as an antioxidant to protect your brain against free radicals.

The *Journal of Neuroscience* has published other studies of middle-aged rats fed diets with added spinach, strawberry extract, or vitamin E. After 9 months, they found that spinach proved to be the most potent at protecting nerve cells in two parts of the brain against the effects of aging.

While spinach contains particularly high levels of polyphenols, it isn't the only green vegetable with high amounts of this phytonutrient group. Other green veggies also contain high levels and are excellent choices for protecting your brain against disease.

How to Benefit

You may be wondering how to get more spinach into your diet, particularly if you're not a fan of it. Fortunately, you can forget what you may have felt about spinach in the past and start to enjoy it today. Here are some of my favorite ways to enjoy this brain-boosting superfood.

- Enjoy a spinach or arugula salad with your favorite cooked or raw mushrooms, hard-boiled egg, and raw cashews. Top it with a delicious salad dressing, such as one of the many recipes included in Part III of this book.

- Add a handful of raw spinach or other leafy greens, such as spring mix or kale, to your morning or afternoon fruit smoothie. It adds a powerful punch of nutrients without changing the taste too much. The color may look less than appetizing, but the flavor will be masked by the fruit.

- Lightly sauté spinach, kale, or collard greens in a little olive oil with some freshly minced garlic. Remove from the heat and toss with a little fresh lemon juice. Even clients who can't stand cooked greens frequently tell me how much they enjoy them prepared this way.

Super Health Bonus

Spinach and other leafy greens are also packed with vitamin A, which helps maintain healthy eyes and vision. I've had numerous clients report an improvement in night vision after they started eating spinach on a regular basis. Leafy greens also contain high amounts of alpha lipoic acid—one of the best defenders of brain health and fighters of fatigue. Alpha lipoic acid protects the energy centers of your cells to ensure that they remain intact for optimum energy production. You can thank lipoic acid for the energy boost you'll likely feel when you make leafy greens a regular part of your diet.

60-SECOND BRAIN HEALTH TIP #25:
Opt for Olives to Protect Your Brain

Olives and olive oil give your brain an important omega-9 boost.

The exotic names of olives—Moroccan, kalamata, niçoise, picholine, and Manzanilla—sound almost as good as these varieties of olives taste. But taste is only one of the reasons to enjoy them. Olives are an excellent source of healthy monounsaturated fats and vitamin E. Monounsaturated fats have a beneficial role to play in maintaining the outer membranes of brain cells and protecting your body's genetic material and the energy-producing cellular components (mitochondria) that help fuel your brain.

Vitamin E offers antioxidant protection to the fatty components of your brain and can lower your risk of damage and inflammation. This vitamin is also your body's primary fat-soluble antioxidant, meaning that it neutralizes damaging free radicals in all the fat-rich areas of your body, including your brain and the protective coating of your nerves. And you may recall from an earlier discussion that more than 60 percent of your brain is fat, making vitamin E a significant contributor to brain health. Like other types of mono-unsaturated fats, vitamin E also helps protect the energy production centers in your cells to ensure that your cells are capable of creating adequate energy for your many bodily processes and brain functions.

Olives also help prevent the oxidation of cholesterol. Oxidized cholesterol has been linked to stroke. The anti-inflammatory actions of monounsaturated fats, vitamin E, and beneficial plant chemicals called polyphenols help lessen the likelihood of inflammation in your brain. Olive oil is also rich in omega-9 fatty acids, which are important to your brain.

Because olive oil is extracted from olives, it has the same beneficial properties as olives. However, be sure to use only organic, cold-pressed, extra-virgin olive oil, since it retains more beneficial nutrients and lacks potentially brain-damaging pesticides.

How to Benefit

When cooking with any type of oil, including olive oil, it is important to be sure that the oil never smokes. If it does, it has reached the oil's "smoke point," which is different for every type of oil. The smoke point is the point at which the oil will have a damaging effect on your body. Most types of vegetable oils available in grocery stores are heated to over 500°F during processing, which is well beyond the smoke point even before they get to your kitchen. That means they should be completely avoided. Extra-virgin olive oil is the rare exception that tends to be processed at lower temperatures and is therefore fine for cooking at low temperatures. Remember this when you're cooking with any type of oil: If it smokes while you are heating it, it is essential that you throw it out and start over. Otherwise, the benefits of the oil are destroyed by the heat and it becomes capable of damaging cells in your brain through free radicals and inflammatory processes. Also, be sure to choose olives that are free from sulfites, as many commercial brands contain these and other chemical preservatives.

Super Health Bonus

In addition to protecting against brain disease, vitamin E works as a powerful antioxidant that reduces the damage caused by pollutants. It may also protect against colon cancer.

60-SECOND BRAIN HEALTH TIP #26:
Reap Rosemary for Brain Health Rewards

Research shows that rosemary is valuable for the prevention and treatment of dementia.

Not just great for meat dishes, now there are more reasons than ever before to enjoy rosemary and the brain health benefits this fragrant herb offers.

I keep a rosemary topiary in a pot at my front door. Because its fragrant aroma is absolutely delightful, I frequently run my hands through its branches to send the smell wafting through the air. Rosemary's name, *Rosmarinus officinalis*, means "dew of the sea," which is probably linked to its native region—the Mediterranean. Rosemary has been used in many cultures as a symbol for remembering those who have passed away; sprigs of the herb are placed on coffins or tombstones. It is cited in Shakespearean literature when Ophelia petitions Hamlet with, "There's rosemary, that's for remembrance. Pray you love, remember." This is a reference to rosemary's long-standing reputation for enhancing memory. In ancient Greece, students inserted rosemary sprigs into their hair when studying for exams.

Rosemary's reputation for enhancing memory likely stems from its research-proven ability to increase blood flow to the brain, thereby improving concentration.[44] Other research proves that rosemary's reputation as a memory aid is well deserved. Researchers at Poland's Department of Pharmaceutical Botany and Plant Biotechnology at Poznan University of Medical Sciences found that when rosemary is eaten as part of a regular diet or used as a natural medicine, it has the ability to improve long-term memory in animals. The scientists found that rosemary slowed the degradation of an important brain hormone known as acetylcholine. Acetylcholine is involved in the formation of new memories and the regulation of muscle activity. The researchers propose that rosemary may be valuable for the prevention and treatment of dementia.[45]

Other research shows that rosemary has anti-inflammatory effects and holds promise as a natural remedy for atherosclerosis—a chronic inflammatory condition that leads to stroke. Based on their positive findings, the scientists anticipate that rosemary has the potential to be developed into a natural anti-atherosclerosis medication or functional food.[46]

How to Benefit

This pine-like herb does more than spice up a roast of beef; it also offers anti-inflammatory protection to the delicate human brain. Add finely chopped rosemary to bread, buns, or savory baked goods. Rosemary is a delicious addition to chicken, lamb, and beef, as well as to omelets and tomato sauces, although I hope you'll be cutting back on red meat. It can be pureed with olive oil to make a delicious dipping oil to use on your bread in place of butter. Or you can make rosemary tea: Add 2 teaspoons of dried rosemary needles or a 4-inch sprig of fresh rosemary to boiled water and let it steep for 10 minutes. Strain and drink.

Super Health Bonus

Rosemary can help thinning hair regrow. In the journal *Phytotherapy Research*, scientists found that applying an extract made of rosemary leaves improved hair regrowth in animals affected by excess amounts of the hormone testosterone. Both men and women can have excess amounts of testosterone, which can cause hair thinning. Scientists found that the rosemary extract appears to block dihydrotestosterone, the active form of testosterone, from binding to androgen receptor sites.[47] Research also found that supplementation with a standardized extract of carnosic acid—one of rosemary's active ingredients—demonstrated the ability to target prostate cancer cells, as opposed to "normal" cells.[48] This study suggests the promise of a rosemary-based, all-natural cancer prevention aid.

60-SECOND BRAIN HEALTH TIP #27:
Regularly Enjoy Tomatoes for a Sharper Memory

Lycopene found in tomatoes significantly cuts stroke risk.

If you're only enjoying tomatoes as part of an occasional pasta dinner, you might want to expand your tomato repertoire. That's because more and more research is showing that tomatoes are great for your health, including the health of your brain.

In an important study known as the Nun Study, scientists at the University of Kentucky studied the effects of lycopene, one of the naturally present compounds in tomatoes, on a group of nuns. They found improved physical abilities and sharper memories in those with the highest amounts in their diets.

Lycopene has also been found to reduce the risk of heart disease and stroke. Research shows that the lycopene found in tomatoes, when eaten regularly, can reduce your risk of heart disease by 29 percent. Fresh tomatoes and tomato extracts have been shown in research to lower total cholesterol, LDL cholesterol, and triglycerides. They have also been shown to prevent clumping in the blood (known as platelet aggregation), which is a risk factor for atherosclerosis and stroke. Additionally, research in the journal *Harvard Health Letter* found that diets rich in tomatoes can help prevent stroke. The scientists chalk up the results to tomatoes' rich lycopene content.[49]

As if that weren't enough reason to eat more tomatoes, plenty of research shows that lycopene is a powerful antioxidant that helps destroy brain-damaging free radicals. Lycopene even protects your genetic material against damage and the resulting disease.

How to Benefit

Tomatoes are delicious and so versatile. They can be enjoyed in pasta, salads, soups, stews, wraps, curries, and many of your favorite dishes.

Some people claim that tomatoes should be eaten cooked, for maximum nutritional value. But that's not the full story. While lycopene is best absorbed from cooked tomatoes, vitamin C and the enzymes found in tomatoes are most beneficial if eaten uncooked. So I suggest mixing things up a bit. Relish cooked tomatoes in soups, stews, and curries. Enjoy raw ones in salads, sandwiches, and salsas. Research also shows that the form of lycopene found in yellow and orange tomatoes is better absorbed than that found in red tomatoes. That doesn't mean you can't enjoy the red ones, but throw some multicolor heirloom tomatoes into the mix, too.

Super Health Bonus

Because tomatoes are also a rich source of the phytonutrients beta-carotene, lutein, and zeaxanthin, they can help improve vision and protect your eyes from degeneration. And tomatoes' lycopene content will give your body a boost in the prevention of cancer.

60-SECOND BRAIN HEALTH TIP #28:
Rev Up Your Brain with Resveratrol

Resveratrol, found in grapes, protects brain cells from damage while helping to prevent Alzheimer's disease.

The compound known as resveratrol, which is found in purple and red grapes, offers this impressive brain protection. Produced by grapevines, resveratrol appears to be the plants' first line of defense against stress, injury, and infection. Once we eat these delightful fruits, they confer their beneficial healing effects on us.

Research by Dr. Egemen Savaskan at the University of Basel, in Switzerland, found that resveratrol helps protect brain cells from damage from the beta-amyloid plaques linked with Alzheimer's disease and dementia.[50] The study found that resveratrol mops up free radicals and protects brain cells from plaque buildup. Dr. Savaskan stresses that his findings suggest that resveratrol may help to protect against Alzheimer's disease.

Resveratrol also appears to work in other ways to improve brain health. Resveratrol has been found to protect the heart and blood vessels against heart disease and therefore may play a protective role in the prevention of stroke. High doses of resveratrol boost blood flow to the brain and slow the effects of aging. Additionally, resveratrol has also been found to reduce inflammation.[51] When it comes to brain health, resveratrol is proving itself invaluable.

How to Benefit

Resveratrol is a naturally occurring substance found in red and purple grapes, grape juice, and red wine. It is a powerful antioxidant that destroys free radicals, seeking them out and eliminating these harmful substances before they can cause damage to your brain. Resveratrol is behind the many articles touting red wine as beneficial for your brain; however, these articles aren't telling the whole story. The alcohol in red wine (and any other type of wine) kills brain cells, so it is best avoided in any brain health plan and should be drunk in moderation only if there is no history of brain disease in your family. Alcohol should especially be avoided by anyone currently suffering from a brain disease. Instead, get your resveratrol from purple or red grapes and purple grape juice.

Grapes are a delicious addition to a leafy green salad and can be blended with oil and vinegar to make a great salad dressing. You can also add them to grain and meat dishes or chop them with some fresh plums and apples to make a sweet chutney to serve alongside curries or fish dishes.

Resveratrol is also found in lower concentrations in blueberries and raspberries. You can also take supplements to obtain higher doses of resveratrol.

The study-proven dose is typically 250 milligrams of resveratrol daily. This amount is almost impossible to obtain from your diet. People already experiencing a serious brain disease may benefit from a higher dose—up to 500 milligrams daily. Of course, if you're taking any supplement, especially in higher doses, you should check with a doctor familiar with resveratrol first.

Super Health Bonus

Resveratrol has also been found to protect against cancer by inhibiting the growth of cancer cells and protecting genetic material from damage.[52] So while you're busy munching on grapes for their brain health benefits, you're also helping to protect yourself against cancer.

60-SECOND BRAIN HEALTH TIP #29:
Take a Coffee Break to Maximize Your Brain Power

Cut your Alzheimer's risk with a daily cup of java.

If you've been feeling guilty about that cup of java, don't. When it comes to brain health, research in the *Journal of the American Medical Association* found that regular coffee consumption lowers your risk of developing Parkinson's disease. And that's not all. In a Florida-based study, researchers found that women who drank 3 cups of coffee daily had a reduced risk of Alzheimer's disease.[53]

So how does coffee work to prevent brain diseases? According to an animal study, researchers found that caffeine supplementation, combined with moderate swimming, reduced inflammation.[54] And further research supports the caffeine–inflammation reduction hypothesis. A study at the University of Illinois found that caffeine may block brain inflammation linked with brain diseases.[55]

How to Benefit

You might think that benefiting from coffee consumption is fairly obvious. After all, most North Americans drink coffee, so it should be straightforward.

But not everyone should drink coffee. Ditch the coffee (and caffeine in general) if you are pregnant or nursing. There's controversy over caffeine consumption during pregnancy, so staying away from the java while pregnant may be a good idea. In a study of children born to pregnant women who ingested caffeine, the caffeine-exposed babies had signs of impaired growth, including low birth weight.[56]

Pregnant and nursing women aren't the only ones who should stay clear of coffee. Women at risk of diabetes, you might also want to skip the coffee.[57] Scientists studying the way caffeine affects people made an interesting discovery: Higher caffeine consumption was associated with a *decreased* risk of diabetes in men but an *increased* risk in women.[58]

How much coffee or caffeine is too much? Everyone is different and has a different caffeine tolerance. One person's perfect amount is another person's nerve-rattling, hand-shaking, can't-sleep-at-night amount. What's right for you depends on many factors, including whether you metabolize caffeine slowly (it stays in your system longer), whether you're on medications that slow your rate of caffeine metabolism (such as the birth control pill, which tends to double your jolt), and whether you suffer from a nervous system disorder or insomnia. So pay attention to your body and cut back if you have trouble sleeping or feel shaky or irritable.

So exactly how much caffeine are you getting? The average person consumes 300 milligrams (mg) of caffeine, which most doctors consider moderate consumption. Anything above 300 mg daily is considered excessive. Keep in mind that every cup of coffee and tea contains a different amount of caffeine. Starbucks coffee, for example, tends to contain about 20 mg of caffeine per ounce, so a 16-ounce coffee provides 320 mg, which is more than the average daily amount, while another coffee company's product is likely to have less than that.[59] You might also be inclined to think that decaffeinated coffee is free of caffeine, but that's just not the case. Decaf coffee still contains some caffeine. It is simply caffeinated coffee that is processed to remove a large percentage of the caffeine.

On its own, coffee is packed with health-giving antioxidants, but it's rarely the health drink it could be, thanks to the ways most people customize it. The same is true for tea. There are many ways you can help ensure that your coffee habit is a healthy one. Here are eight simple ways to make your coffee (or tea) a brain-healthy and planet-friendly option.

1. **Choose organic coffee or tea.** Both crops tend to be heavily sprayed with pesticides (sometimes ones that are banned in North America but legal in the countries where these crops are grown), so you may be getting more than just coffee or tea when you select anything but organic.

2. **Choose fair trade for a healthy conscience.** Coffee is big business. According to the United Nations, it is the second most widely traded commodity (after oil). As such, its growth and harvesting are subjected to a wide variety of exploitive labor conditions, including child labor, in some countries.[60]

3. **Skip the sugar.** Or if you must have it, select a sweetener such as organic coconut sugar, which has fewer grams of sugar (3 grams) than white or brown sugar (4 grams). It doesn't sound like a big difference, but over time that means you'll have cut your sugar consumption by 25 percent with almost no effort. Coconut sugar contains chromium and other natural minerals that aid sugar metabolism in your body. Better yet, use the natural herb stevia, which contains no sugar and is a brain-healthy option. (See 60-Second Brain Health Tip #1 on page 49 for more information about stevia.)

4. **Pass on the flavored syrups.** Most are made with high fructose corn syrup, which has been linked to weight gain and obesity. They also contain artificial flavors and preservatives, such as potassium sorbate and sodium benzoate. Potassium sorbate has been shown in human studies to be both genotoxic and mutagenic.[61] That means it damages genetic material and can cause mutations linked to disease. Sodium benzoate converts to the carcinogen benzene in your body.

5. **Say sayonara to sugar-free syrups and artificial sweeteners.** If you're thinking that you're safe because you only use sugar-free syrups and artificial sweeteners, think again. Not only do these syrups usually contain the above-mentioned preservatives, but they also typically contain one of the following synthetic sweeteners: Splenda, Sweet'N Low, or AminoSweet. Contrary to claims that Splenda is a sugar substitute suitable for weight loss, it (sucralose) was shown by Duke University scientists to *increase* body weight, be absorbed by fat cells, and reduce beneficial intestinal flora by 50 percent, which further contributes to inflammatory illnesses—including brain diseases. Sweet'NLow (saccharin) is a coal tar derivative that has been linked to breathing difficulties, headaches, skin eruptions, and diarrhea. AminoSweet (the new name for aspartame) has been linked to an enormous list of health conditions, including brain tumors, depression, headaches and migraines, joint pain, chronic fatigue, and more.

6. **Skip the whip.** Adding whipped cream to your coffee adds about 100 calories to each drink. That's an extra 36,500 calories a year if you only drink one a day. And you may recall our earlier discussion about dairy products and the negative impact they can have on your brain and overall health.

7. **Pick milk alternatives over cow's milk.** If you're going to add milk to your coffee, it's best to pick almond, rice, or organic soy (other soy is genetically modified) milk. Cow's milk is not the health food the dairy bureaus would have us believe it is.

8. **Definitely skip the coffee whitener.** It is made from corn syrup solids, which are almost always genetically modified and which typically contain brain-damaging trans fats. The companies that make them are not required to report the trans fats because the serving size is so small, but it adds up to a lot of trans fats when you drink this stuff a few times a day, every day.

Super Health Bonus

Coffee consumption may help protect against cancer. Women who drank 4 cups of coffee daily had a 25 percent reduction in endometrial cancer.[62] In another study, mice fed caffeine developed 27 percent fewer skin cancer growths after UV exposure. Combining the caffeine with exercise resulted in a 62 percent reduction in tumors.[63] The researchers believe the results will translate to people, as well.

60-SECOND BRAIN HEALTH TIP #30:
Take a Pit Stop on the Road to Brain Health

Apricots, peaches, cherries, and plums protect both the watery and fatty parts of your brain from damage.

Take a pit stop for brain health—by eating fruits with pits, that is. Research shows that fruits that contain pits are among those with the highest concentrations of nutritional compounds called flavonoids, which protect and heal your brain. That includes apricots, peaches, cherries, and plums.

Fruits that are blue, red, or purple contain a special group of flavonoids called proanthocyanidins, which protect both the watery and fatty parts of your brain against free radical damage. They seem to stop free radicals in their tracks, making these foods especially valuable in the prevention of brain disease. Plums and cherries are among the foods with the highest concentrations of these potent antioxidants. To learn more about cherries, see 60-Second Brain Health Tip #12 on page 87.

How to Benefit

Eat at least one pit-containing fruit every day. In addition to fresh apricots, peaches, cherries, and plums, you can enjoy dried fruits that once contained pits to take advantage of the many brain-healing flavonoids they contain. These include dried apricots, prunes, cherries, and peaches. If you're eating dried fruits, be sure they are sulfite-free and unsweetened. Many dried fruits are pretreated with sugar and sulfites, neither of which is good for your brain. Dried fruits that lack both sugar and sulfites are often slightly browner than their chemically treated counterparts. Don't worry about the color; these fruits are nutritionally superior and better for your brain.

Super Health Bonus

In addition to protecting your brain against inflammation and disease, pro-anthocyanidin-rich fruits such as plums, prunes, and cherries reduce other effects of aging and inflammation while also helping with weight loss in those who are overweight. You may notice an improvement in your allergies, too, since they contain a protein with anti-allergic effects. Peaches and apricots are also high in alpha- and beta-carotenes, which boost your immunity and protect your eyesight.

60-SECOND BRAIN HEALTH TIP #31:
Get Teary-Eyed to Transform Your Brain Health

Onions and garlic contain powerful natural substances that protect your brain against damaging plaques linked to brain diseases.

General Ulysses S. Grant once stated, "I will not move my army without onions." Perhaps he understood the food's potent medicinal properties. Regular consumption of onions, which is described as two or more times per week, has been associated with lower cholesterol levels and reduced blood pressure (when it is high), both of which help reduce your risk of stroke, among other diseases.[64]

The beneficial effects may be associated with the sulfur compounds found in onions, as well as vitamin B_6 and the mineral chromium; all of these help reduce high levels of homocysteine, a risk factor for stroke and inflammation. Your liver needs the sulfur compounds to eliminate the by-products of inflammation and potentially brain-damaging environmental or food toxins to which you're exposed. Onions also contain vitamin C, quercetin, and phytochemicals called isothiocyanates, which help to alleviate inflammation.

Onions aren't the only sulfur-containing foods that can boost your brain health. Garlic's pungent aroma, potent flavor, and powerful medicinal qualities also make it a great choice for your brain-boosting diet. Garlic may be the original wonder drug. Remains of the plant have been found in caves used by humans 10,000 years ago, and a Sumerian clay tablet dated from 3000 BC contains a chiseled prescription for garlic.[65] Supplements of a 2 percent standardized potency of aged garlic extract (AGE) were shown in research published in the *Journal of Ethnopharmacology* to be beneficial in reducing both brain inflammation and amyloid plaques linked to Alzheimer's disease.[66] Another study in the journal *Phytotherapy Research* found that AGE prevented the deterioration of memory and memory-related tasks in animals.[67]

Both onions and garlic contain compounds that inhibit lipoxygenase and cyclooxygenase (the enzymes that generate inflammatory substances) and reduce inflammation.

How to Benefit

There are very few savory dishes that won't benefit from the addition of garlic or onions. Cooking or roasting garlic and onions helps to mellow both their flavors and aromas; use raw or roasted to enhance soups, stews, stir-fries, curries, sauces, and pastas. They are staples in many European and Asian cuisines and are popular in North America, as well. The proliferation of garlic-themed restaurants and food shops is a testament to garlic's diverse and delicious contribution to our diet. Additionally, you may wish to supplement with AGE to obtain the study-proven brain health benefits discussed above. Take a 2 percent standardized potency of AGE. Follow the dosage directions on the package.

Super Health Bonus

Garlic and onions help to regulate cholesterol levels, reducing your risk of heart disease. They are also potent antimicrobials that may help reduce the frequency with which you experience colds or flu.

Brain Books in Action

NAME: Renee Carter

AGE: 36

OCCUPATION: Office administrator

"Since following this program, my visualization skills, vocabulary, and long-term memory have become clearer. I feel like my digestion has improved, and losing almost 8 pounds has been a very nice 'side effect.'"

How I Got Here: When Renee Carter became a new mother, she understood that some degree of distraction and forgetfulness would be normal. However, when she found herself forgetting what she was saying midsentence and unable to recall what she had said 20 minutes ago, she became worried. "When I started putting files in the wrong place at work, I knew I needed to see a doctor."

Just 2 days after sharing her health concerns with her husband, Renee learned about the 60 Seconds to Boost Your Brain Power Health Challenge and decided to give the program a try.

Progress Report: Within a week of starting the plan, Renee's brain fog lifted and she felt much more energetic and positive about her life. "I was driving to work and a warm, thankful feeling washed over me. I didn't feel so overwhelmed. I felt calm and focused."

Gone were the processed, sugary foods she had been eating every day. Instead, Renee enjoyed easy-to-follow, delicious recipes that were budget-friendly, too. "My joints and muscles stopped aching, and I felt the urge to draw, an activity that had once been my passion."

Renee also noticed that her newfound attitude about exercise made it easier to fit into her schedule. "I've started to make time to exercise, and while it's not as often as I'd like, I'm more accepting of my pace; I've learned that placing unrealistic expectations on myself leads to disappointment, irritability, anger, and stress." Instead, Renee tries to focus on doing what she can, when she can.

Beyond: Given the positive results of her new approach to living, Renee decided to stick with the nutrition and exercise program she started. "I've learned that technology, food, family, finances, and lack of exercise all have negative effects that can cause brain function to decline. In learning more about how my brain works, I've definitely learned to nurture it better nutritionally and allow it more downtime to reenergize!"

CHAPTER 5

WEEK 3: STRATEGIZE

Adopt These Tips and Tricks to Boost Your Brain and Memory Power

This week I will introduce you to the best brain-supporting strategies to boost your memory and brain health. You'll discover the best lifestyle changes and additions to make to keep a healthy brain for life. Most of these strategies take a minute or less to implement and provide years of brain power. You learned about the benefits of exercise in Chapter 2, but you'll learn about many other brain boosters here. Choose a minimum of two tips from this chapter to include in your life, but feel free to add more if you'd like. The more, the better. And as you'll soon discover, these brain-boosting strategies are simpler than you might think to incorporate into your life.

In this section, you'll learn to:

42. Walk Your Way to a Bigger, Better Brain (page 152)

   A *daily walk can stave off dementia.*

43. Practice Mind over Platter Because Portion Size Matters (page 155)

   Kick the overeating habit to significantly reduce memory loss and cognitive impairment.

60-SECOND BRAIN HEALTH TIP #32:
Sleep Your Way to a Super Brain

Get at least 8 hours of sleep to boost your creative juices.

Seriously, you can sleep your way to a healthier brain . . . and that's a strategy even couch potatoes can appreciate. According to new research at the University of Notre Dame and Boston College, getting at least 8 hours of sleep helps your brain to think more creatively. The scientists also found that people who get more sleep are better able to organize memories and reconfigure them in a way that produces new insights and creative ideas. From this study, researchers determined that sleep helps consolidate memories, fixing them in your brain so you can retrieve them later.[1]

Other research shows that not getting enough sleep on a regular basis is a recipe for memory disaster. According to sleep expert and author of *The Promise of Sleep*, William C. Dement, MD, PhD, we need at least 7 to 8 hours of sleep per night. Dr. Dement also found that your body keeps track of a sleep debt. If you don't get sufficient sleep on a regular basis, it is comparable to making ongoing withdrawals from a sleep account. We need to make up the lost hours soon afterward or our sleep account continues to go further and further into debt.

How to Benefit

So how exactly do you reap the rewards of sleep if you're having trouble getting to sleep or staying asleep, or if you experience restless sleep? Here are some of my favorite sleep-improving strategies.

- Avoid eating for at least 3 hours before bed, as indigestion, bloating, or heartburn can interfere with your ability to fall asleep. Definitely skip the caffeine in the evening or anytime after 3:00 p.m. if you have difficulty sleeping.

- Get into a regular evening relaxation ritual: Dim the lights, stop working, take a bath, or do something relaxing before bedtime. Once you've made this a habit, your body will naturally start preparing you for sleep when you begin your routine, and over time, getting a good night's sleep will become easier.

- Unplug electronic devices and blue light–emitting appliances such as televisions, smartphones, computers, etc., because the blue light can interfere with your sleep cycles. If you need a night light, choose a red bulb; red light doesn't seem to interfere with the body's ability to fall into a state of deep sleep.

- Go to sleep at the same time each night. Your body will start to adjust to these patterns, helping you feel sleepy when your bedtime approaches.

- Alan Hirsch, MD, author of *Life's a Smelling Success*, found that smelling pure lavender calmed the entire nervous system in only a minute, helping people to feel more relaxed and sleepier. Sniff some lavender essential oil or flowers, or spray lavender water on your pillowcase (water only, because the oil may stain). Be sure to choose organic lavender oil, not fragrance oil, since the latter has no health benefits and frequently contains toxic substances.

Super Health Bonus

Getting more sleep helps you lose weight if you are overweight. That's because sleep-deprived individuals experience six barriers to weight loss, according to research: They are more likely to experience intense sweet cravings; are less likely to feel full, even after eating a lot of food; are more prone to compulsive overeating; have a tendency toward lean muscle loss; exercise less; and experience an impaired ability to burn carbohydrates. Ensuring adequate time for sleep is a simple way to help balance your weight and experience better health. Additional research shows that sleep deprivation slows the rate at which you burn fat. Researchers at the University of Chicago discovered that well-rested women had faster metabolic rates and ate 15 percent less food than women who didn't get sufficient sleep. So don't be surprised if you boost your brain health and lose a few pounds after making an effort to get more sleep.

60-SECOND BRAIN HEALTH TIP #33:
Use It or Lose It to Supercharge Your Memory

Challenge your mind to boost connections between brain cells and boost memory.

More and more research shows that, similar to muscles that get out of shape when they're not used regularly, your brain needs to be challenged on a regular basis for optimal performance. Each of your brain cells has a long, wire-like structure called an axon that sends out hormones called neurotransmitters to generate an electrical charge between brain cells. Each of these neurotransmitters performs a different function, depending on what type of message the brain cell is trying to send. Some initiate bodily functions, while others stop the same functions.

Between your brain cells there are tiny gaps, known as synapses, across which the neurotransmitters travel to send their messages. These synapses are constantly changing as a result of feedback from your environment. Over time, some synapses grow stronger through learning, while others weaken or disappear if not used. Your brain recognizes which synapses are needed and which ones have not been used for a while. And if you don't use certain synapses for a period of time, your brain essentially dismantles the connection.

To illustrate your brain's miraculous ability to constantly fine-tune the connections it keeps or loses, let's look at language skills. Remember those second languages we learned in high school? I learned French, but perhaps you learned Spanish, German, or another language. When you start learning a new language, your brain sets up all kinds of synapses linked to languages, but over time, if you don't maintain the new language synapses linked to learning, you may forget what you've learned. That doesn't mean that you can't learn a new language or other skills at some future time, but it will be easier if you continuously use this particular skill set throughout your life.

In a study shared in *Medical News Today,* researcher William Greenough discovered a way to quickly increase the number of connections in animal brains by 25 percent. He simply exposed the animals to what he termed an "enriched environment." He indicates, "What we know from animals suggests that the harder you use your brain, whether it's thinking or exercising, the more in shape it's going to be."[2] His research shows that when we expose ourselves to new intellectual challenges, we don't just have improved mental fitness; our brain actually grows—not in size, but in interconnectedness. It makes it easier for us to make future mental connections.

While there is extensive research to support that educated people have an improved ability to ward off Alzheimer's disease, education alone is not enough to ensure improved brain function. College graduates who have mentally inactive lives have fewer brain synapses than graduates who stay intellectually active. So a college degree does not guarantee immunity to brain diseases or memory loss. And it's certainly not necessary to have a high level of formal education to stay educated. Your formal education is much less important than whether you continue to learn new things throughout your life. Your brain is designed for lifelong learning, and your brain health depends on it. For most of us, that means making some effort to ramp up the intellectual challenges we give our brains.

So when it comes to brushing up on a language, there's no time like the present. And now there's even more reason to do so. A study from the Rotman Research Institute found that bilingual Alzheimer's patients started experiencing symptoms of the disease 5 years later than their unilingual counterparts.[3] When we think in a different language, we reinforce brain connections that we might not otherwise use.

Another study published in the journal *Neurology* reviewed the work histories of people with and without Alzheimer's. The study found that those people who developed the illness had fewer mentally challenging assignments as part of their regular work lives. The researchers found that the more intellectually demanding jobs boosted cognitive reserves and helped to stave off dementia.

How to Benefit

It's time to dust off those language books, head to a new class, call up a friend to play chess, or simply challenge your mind more on the job. There are not only mental health benefits to pushing yourself intellectually, but there are serious brain health advantages, too. There is no limit to the skills you can acquire. Set some new intellectual goals and begin today to work toward achieving them.

Super Health Bonus

Learning new skills often means meeting new people, and more and more research links improved overall health and happiness with a strong social support system.

60-SECOND BRAIN HEALTH TIP #34:

Knock Out Infection with a Natural Antibacterial Punch

Add a natural antibiotic to knock out brain-damaging Helicobacter pylori *infections.*

When it comes to our brain health, memory, and cognitive function, few people think of infections. Conversely, when we think of the infectious bacteria *Helicobacter pylori* (*H. pylori*), people who are familiar with the bacteria think of ulcers. But more and more research links this menacing microbe with poor mental function, dementia, and even Alzheimer's disease.[4]

Research published in the journal *Helicobacter* found that *H. pylori* produces a low-grade inflammatory state within the body, which can be a precursor to many potential illnesses, including brain diseases.[5] Additionally, the study showed that the bacteria mimics the body's own molecular functions and interferes with the absorption of nutrients, particularly vitamin B_{12}, which is necessary for the production of neurotransmitters (including serotonin, dopamine, and acetylcholine) that allow nerve cells to transmit memory signals. Research links a vitamin B_{12} deficiency to an increased risk of Alzheimer's disease and dementia.[6] Vitamin B_{12} deficiencies are also linked to depression and poor memory.[7, 8, 9] For more information about vitamin B_{12}, its role in brain health, and how to restore your B_{12} levels, check out 60-Second Brain Health Tip #45 on page 165. It's equally important to address any underlying *H. pylori* infection.

How to Benefit

To find out if you have an *H. pylori* infection, ask your doctor to conduct laboratory testing. A urea breath test determines whether you have a stomach or duodenum infection. A blood antibody test determines whether your immune system has made substances (antibodies) in an effort to fight an *H. pylori* infection. It indicates whether you currently have or have had an *H. pylori* infection in the past. A stool antigen test is another laboratory test used to detect past or present *H. pylori* infections. It determines whether there are immune substances in your intestines that indicate an encounter with *H. pylori*.[10] Ask your doctor to conduct the relevant tests for you.

If your doctor determines that you have an *H. pylori* infection, it is important to address it immediately. *H. pylori* infections are often linked to overuse of nonsteroidal anti-inflammatory drugs (NSAIDs), which are available over-the-counter.[11] So one of the first steps is to stop using NSAIDs, including Tylenol, Advil, and other common pain medications. Doing so won't kill the infection, but it will at least stop damaging your gut lining. Once your gut lining is damaged, bacteria can hijack your body's nutrient absorption system via your gut to gain direct access to your bloodstream.

Next, it is important to start using proven natural medicines to treat the infection. While many doctors prescribe antibiotics, *H. pylori* is becoming increasingly resistant to antibiotic drugs. That means these drugs will have limited, if any, effectiveness in eliminating the infection.

Certain probiotics have shown great promise in the treatment of *H. pylori*. But not just any probiotic supplement will do. Most strains of probiotics are not effective against *H. pylori*, so it is imperative that you choose one that has a proven track record of killing *H. pylori*. If you choose to take antibiotic drugs, a Russian study found that the probiotic *Bifidobacteria bifiform*, taken along with the standard drug treatment for *H. pylori*, improved the effectiveness of the drug treatment while also reducing the side effects of the drugs. The Russian scientists also found that the probiotics demonstrated antibacterial action and enhanced the body's own immune response against *H. pylori*.[12] Whereas the probiotics were used as an adjunct to drug treatment, the probiotics were effective against the condition when taken on their own, as well.

Bifidobacteria bifiform has a proven track record of treating *H. pylori*, but it isn't the only probiotic that can.[13] Additional research shows that specific strains of probiotics also have the ability to treat *H. pylori* infections on their own. In other studies, scientists found that either *Lactobacillus* strains on their own or in combination with *Bifidobacterium* and *Saccharomyces* species effectively reduced the symptoms of *H. pylori* infections.[14] If you're using antibiotic treatments, it is best to add a probiotic supplement with these above-mentioned strains for greater effectiveness against *H. pylori* infections.

Once you've selected a probiotic supplement that includes strains that have a proven track record against this infection, it is important to add other remedies that boost the probiotic's effectiveness or assist in killing *H. pylori*.

Naturally occurring compounds found in cranberry juice have been shown in many studies to be effective against *H. pylori* infections. Researchers conducted a study at the Laboratory of Microbiology and Probiotics, Institute of Nutrition and Food Technology, University of Chile, in Santiago, Chile, to assess the possible effects of combining cranberry juice with probiotics to treat *H. pylori* infections. The study showed the promise of treating *H. pylori* with a combination therapy of cranberry juice and *L. johnsonii La1* probiotics.[15] At the time of writing this book, the probiotic strains *L. johnsonii La1*, *L. reuteri*, and *S. boulardii* have shown the greatest effectiveness against *H. pylori* when combined with cranberry juice. Drink 8 ounces of unsweetened cranberry juice daily for at least 1 month. Ideally, dilute the cranberry juice 1:1 in water, as well. Don't skip any days. If you miss a day, begin again to take cranberry juice for a minimum of 1 full month.

Oregano oil has demonstrated significant effectiveness against *H. pylori* infections on its own, but it usually works most effectively when taken with other antibacterial remedies, because they tend to have synergistic effects. Oregano oil taken on a daily basis has demonstrated significant effectiveness against *H. pylori* when it's taken in combination with pure, unsweetened cranberry juice.[16] Oregano oil supplements vary widely in quality and effectiveness. Choose an undiluted, high-potency product, such as North American Herb & Spice company's Physician's Strength Wild Oregano Oil, which is available in drops and in gel capsules through your natural physician. If you can't find one who sells this high-potency product, the company also sells a wild oregano oil that is available to the public. Take two gel capsules three times daily for at least 1 month.

According to research presented in the *World Journal of Gastroenterology*, of the 25 remedies tested by the authors of the study, turmeric is the most effective natural remedy against *H. pylori* infections.[17] Choose a high-potency turmeric supplement with a standardized extract of curcumin, one of the effective ingredients against infections.

Super Health Bonus

In addition to their proven effectiveness against *H. pylori* infections, the probiotic strains mentioned above, unsweetened cranberry juice, oregano oil, and turmeric have all demonstrated effectiveness against many other types of infections, so you will likely see a boost in your immunity to infectious illnesses.

60-SECOND BRAIN HEALTH TIP #35:

Take the Road Less Traveled to Build New Brain Connections

Try something new to build new brain connections and boost memory.

We are creatures of habit. We usually take the same route to and from work. We frequently eat the same 10 or 20 foods on a regular basis. We watch the same television shows every week. We use the same household products and shop in the same stores. We go to the same coffee shops or restaurants.

The simple act of trying new things or taking a different route home from work actually strengthens the connections between brain cells or builds new connections in your brain. This doesn't have to mean something extreme, like base jumping or rock climbing; simple things, like cooking something different for dinner, talking with new people, going to a gallery, or taking a class to learn a new skill all build new pathways in your brain to improve memory.

How to Benefit

It might not seem like a big deal to take a different route to work or to try new restaurants, but it is a big deal to your brain. It forces your brain to get off autopilot and think about the things you do on a regular basis. Every day, ask yourself if you can do things you normally do a bit differently than you've done them in the past. It could be as simple as striking up a conversation with someone new or taking the scenic route to work, but it all helps boost your brain health.

Super Health Bonus

Trying new things boosts your brain connections and brain health, but it also gives you the opportunity to discover new foods you might love, meet new people who might become friends, or simply expose your mind to different ideas and ways of thinking. In the process, you may learn new things about yourself and expand your horizons at the same time.

60-SECOND BRAIN HEALTH TIP #36:
Beat Stress Before It Affects Your Brain

Soothe stress and boost brain health with seven simple stress-busters.

Stress can cause a significant decline in energy available for your brain, particularly if the stress is chronic or if you have been leading a stressful life for an extended period of time. This can result in memory loss. That's because stress signals your adrenal glands, two triangular-shaped glands that sit atop your kidneys, to release powerful hormones. These hormones reduce the capacity of your brain to utilize glucose (sugar) as energy. When stress becomes chronic, this ongoing release of hormones actually starves your brain of its fuel and lessens brain energy. One of the most immediate symptoms is memory loss or impaired memory. If the stress continues for long periods of time, these stress hormones can even sever important connections between your brain cells. Whatever information may have existed at that connection may be lost. So you can probably understand why stress management is so critical to a healthy brain.

There are many ways to control stress in your life. Everyone experiences stress to some degree or another, but the way in which you choose to deal with it can determine its effects on your body and brain. The most stressed-out people usually don't realize how poorly they are dealing with (or, more aptly, *not* dealing with) stress. Usually these people think they are completely on top of everything in their lives, juggling a hectic work schedule, partner, children and their many activities, family members, in-laws, outlaws, social activities . . . but just thinking about their lives and the mental "to-do" lists they create for themselves is exhausting.

While you may feel that society demands nothing less than constant work and an active social life, your brain may need a pace that is more manageable. Dare I say we may even need to slow down? Sometimes that's just what is necessary to manage stress better: Create fewer time commitments. Alternatively, make a commitment to you, your relaxation, and your brain health.

One of the easiest and cheapest options is to simply take time out to do nothing: no work, no socializing, no television. (As brainless as TV often is, you still need a break from it.) Just be. You may be scoffing, "But I can't. I'm just too busy." If that, or something similar, was your response, you are probably one of the people most in need of slowing down for a bit. If you can't take a brief time-out for your health, then that speaks volumes about the stress of your life.

It's too easy to get caught up in the stresses in life and to put ourselves and our health needs last, but it is important to start considering the long-term effects of doing so. Make your brain health a priority today and every day by making some simple changes in your life.

How to Benefit

Here are eight ways to cope with stress.

1. **Don't skip meals.** Skipping meals when you're busy is a recipe for blood sugar fluctuations. As you just learned, your brain needs a steady supply of energy to function at its best. If you don't have time for meals, just bring a bag of raw, unsalted pumpkin seeds, walnuts, or almonds along and eat a handful or two every 2 to 3 hours to stabilize your blood sugar and brain energy.

2. **Drink water to combat dehydration.** Drink plenty of water throughout the day. Your brain and nerve cells require adequate water to function properly and even to transmit the electrical impulses they use to communicate.

3. **Pop a B complex and some vitamin C.** B-complex vitamins and vitamin C are both depleted by stress. B vitamins are essential for energy production within your body, while vitamin C is the most stress-depleted nutrient.

4. **Give yourself the gift of rest.** Take some time out to replenish and recharge your energy. Enjoy a hot bath, a nap, or a candlelit evening, or head to bed early so you don't wear yourself down during the holidays. A few drops of pure lavender essential oil has been shown to reduce tension and boost relaxation.

5. **It's okay to say no to people who steal your energy and stress you out.** If your heart isn't in it, it's best to honor your instincts and say no.

6. **Live within your means.** Financial stress is damaging to your health, your relationships, and according to new research, even your IQ. Put the credit cards away to avoid overspending.

7. **Go outside and get some fresh air.** Just breathing in some oxygen-rich outdoor air can help reduce stress hormone levels in as little as 1 minute.

8. **Meditate.** Check out 60-Second Brain Health Tip #39 on page 145 to learn how to meditate and take advantage of meditation's stress-busting effects.

Super Health Bonus

Stress aggravates most chronic and acute health conditions, so reducing your stress levels may help with any other health challenges you may be facing.

60-SECOND BRAIN HEALTH TIP #37:
Boost Bacteria to Bolster Your Brain

Give your "second brain" a potent microbial boost to significantly reduce your risk of brain diseases.

Called the "second brain" by leading scientists, a healthy balance of flora in your gut helps to determine whether you'll have a great memory and a strong resistance to brain disease. And what happens in your gut plays a significant role in your brain health. Restoring beneficial bacteria and some healthy yeasts in your intestines can go a long way toward protecting your mental faculties and preventing brain diseases altogether.

When I tell people about this connection between intestinal and brain health—what is known as the gut–brain axis—they frequently tell me that they are covered because they eat yogurt on a regular basis. While yogurt may (or may not) help boost intestinal flora, you need to give your gut a lot more than yogurt to help establish a strong and healthy brain for life. Let's explore some of the exciting research into the link between beneficial microbes in your gut and your overall brain health.

Some probiotics can actually function as antioxidants within your body, reducing the effects of free radical damage and aging, which is especially good news to those seeking to prevent and treat brain diseases. That's because your brain is vulnerable to free radical damage, particularly the 60 percent of your brain that is composed of fat. Probiotics may help to protect the fatty parts of your brain from damage, and this, in turn, may help us prevent serious brain diseases such as Alzheimer's, Parkinson's, dementia, and others.

Swedish researchers found that supplementing with the probiotic strain *Lactobacillus plantarum* resulted in a 37 percent reduction of the chemicals linked to free radical damage that are elevated in patients with many brain and nerve disorders.[18] Additionally, new research at UCLA found that consuming certain strains of probiotics could actually produce many brain health benefits, including improved sensory and emotional processing.[19]

Because your brain plays a significant role in whether you suffer from mental health conditions such as anxiety and depression, it is important to look at cutting-edge research into using probiotics to address these serious health concerns. New research links chronic gastrointestinal disorders to altered behavior and higher rates of anxiety and depression.[20] In animal studies conducted by the Department of Medicine at McMaster University in Canada, the probiotic *Bifidobacterium longum* eliminated anxiety and normalized behavior. It appeared to work by reducing the excitability of the nerves in the gut that connect through the vagus nerve to the central nervous system.[21]

Hungarian researchers found that intestinal inflammation is a key factor in depression and that treating the inflammation with probiotics, along with B-complex vitamins and omega-3 fatty acids, reduced depressive symptoms.[22] See 60-Second Brain Health Tips #45 (page 165) and #22 (page 107) for more information on using these supplements and foods to boost brain health.

Additional French research demonstrates the power of boosting specific strains of probiotics to improve mood and psychological health. They found that healthy study participants experienced reduced psychological stress, depression, anxiety, anger, and hostility, as well as improved problem-solving skills, when taking *Lactobacillus helveticus* and *B. longum* for 30 days.[23]

For more information on the gut–brain axis or body-wide benefits of probiotics, check out my book *The Probiotic Promise*.

How to Benefit

While you can still enjoy yogurt if you are already doing so, please keep in mind that the strains mentioned above are not typically found in yogurt. I'm not aware of any yogurt that contains them. Take a probiotic supplement containing proven strains of brain-boosting probiotics such as *L. plantarum*, *B. longum*, and *L. helveticus* on a daily basis. Store your probiotics in the refrigerator and take them on an empty stomach. (First thing in the morning with a large glass of water tends to work well for most people.)

Additionally, kimchi—the national dish of Korea, which is typically a fermented mixture of cabbage, chiles, and garlic—frequently contains the brain-boosting probiotic strain *L. plantarum*, among many other beneficial microbes. It is an excellent condiment that works well on sandwiches, over brown rice, or as a side dish. Be sure to choose kimchi that hasn't been pasteurized to ensure that the cultures are still intact.

Super Health Bonus

Kimchi is a great all-natural antiviral remedy. New research conducted at the Department of Biology at Georgia State University found that the probiotics in kimchi confer protection against the flu by regulating your body's innate immunity.[24] So if you choose to enjoy kimchi on a regular basis, you'll probably find that you're coming down with fewer flus and viral conditions.

60-SECOND BRAIN HEALTH TIP #38:
Embrace the Tiger and Return to the Mountain for Optimal Brain Health

Stop cognitive decline in its tracks with simple tai chi or qigong exercises.

When I suggest that you embrace the tiger and return to the mountain for brain health, I'm not suggesting that you literally need to hug a large carnivorous predator and leave civilization behind; I'm referring to a tai chi exercise. Not only is tai chi a beautiful and graceful form of exercise, it also offers brain health benefits, according to numerous studies.

Research by Lyvonne Carreiro and her colleagues at the University of Florida found that people experienced less cognitive decline when they incorporated tai chi into their lives. Those people living with Parkinson's disease who attended tai chi classes for only 1 hour weekly for 12 weeks fared better mentally and physically than their counterparts who did not practice tai chi.

Following qigong, another Chinese form of exercise (pronounced chee-GUNG), subjects showed improvement in some aspects of sleep quality. Fatigue remained unchanged in patients with Parkinson's disease.

A study conducted at the University of Bonn, in Germany, explored the effects of qigong. The study involved 56 people suffering from various levels of Parkinson's disease severity. Study participants received 90-minute weekly group instruction for 2 months, followed by a 2-month break and a second 2-month treatment period. Participants were assessed at the beginning of the study and after 3 months, 6 months, and 12 months. Researchers found a significant improvement in the qigong group than in the control group after 3 and 6 months. After 1 year (6 months after the end of the study), there was still a significant and sustained difference between the qigong group and the control group, showing the long-term benefits of qigong exercise in people with Parkinson's disease.[25]

A pilot study published in the *International Journal of Neuroscience* found significant improvements in symptoms of Parkinson's disease sufferers when they engaged in qigong for 6 weeks. They found that following qigong, people showed improvements in sleep quality and significant improvements in gait performance.[26] While the study was small, the results were impressive. And any treatment that shows improvement in Parkinson's disease, particularly one lacking harmful side effects, is worth serious consideration.

Parkinson's disease sufferers aren't the only ones who can benefit from qigong. New research published in the journal *Explore* found that qigong may be helpful in the recovery of people who have suffered a mild traumatic brain injury.[27] (That doesn't mean that it isn't helpful for moderate to severe traumatic brain injury survivors, but rather that this particular study didn't assess qigong with these people.)

How to Benefit

It's easy to start benefiting from tai chi or qigong exercises. Sign up for a local class, pick up an instructional video from your library or online bookstore, or follow along with a book on the topic. Whatever you choose, the brain health rewards will be worth the effort.

Super Health Bonus

Tai chi and qigong exercises were designed to regulate the functions of all the organs and glands in the body. Like many others, you will probably notice improvements in seemingly unrelated health conditions if you stick with these exercises over time.

60-SECOND BRAIN HEALTH TIP #39:
Enjoy the Benefits of Ohm Sweet Ohm

Meditate to quell the brain-damaging effects of stress.

Meditation is quite effective for lessening stress and the resulting stress hormones that have a negative impact on your brain. Many people associate meditation with religion, but it is actually a simple technique that transcends religious beliefs. It is a mental vacation from the stresses of daily life whereby you center your mind and create a sense of peacefulness. The rewards are worth the minimal effort.

In one study published in *Health Behavior News Service*, scientists found that brain scans and blood tests confirmed positive effects of meditation. In this study of 48 employees at a biotechnology company, half were trained in meditation and practiced it for 1 hour a day, 6 days a week, using prerecorded guided meditations. The other half of the participants did not meditate. Dr. Richard J. Davidson at the University of Wisconsin found that the meditators had greater electrical activity in their brains than the nonmeditators. Some of the effects of meditation continued for up to 4 months after the participants discontinued their meditation practice.[28]

Other research shows improvements in mood, pain threshold, immune system activity, and bronchial and arterial smooth muscle tone. The studies also show a decrease in stress hormones and a reversal in the effects of chronic stress.[29]

When we think of things that improve blood flow to the brain, meditation is probably not one of the first things to come to mind. We're far more likely to consider exercises that boost heart rate. But even if you're injured, disabled, or just having trouble exercising, meditation is still an option, as research shows that it improves blood flow to the brain.

Research in *Psychiatry Research* shows that meditation affects the flow of blood to the brain. Scientists at the Ahmanson-Lovelace Brain Mapping Center at UCLA studied the effects of meditation on the "stress" circuits of the brain. Ten experienced meditators performed two types of meditation: a focus-based meditative technique and a breath-based practice. The meditators' brains were scanned using MRI technology before starting, during the meditation practices, and following meditation.

Researchers found that four regions of the brain were affected during meditation and that the two types of meditation states cause different patterns of blood flow to the brain; however, both techniques improved blood flow to the brain. Some of the brain changes continued even after meditation stopped.[30]

While research in this area is still in its infancy, the positive impact of meditation on blood flow to the brain may have applications in treating brain disorders or stroke and in keeping your brain healthy for the long term.

Meditation is simple to learn, requires no expensive equipment, and can be done almost anywhere. All that is needed is a commitment and a small amount of time. While participants in the study mentioned above practiced for 1 hour a day, even a few minutes daily will be helpful.

There are many different types of meditation. Don't get bogged down in finding the ideal one for you; that sort of quest is often just an excuse for procrastinating, anyway. As Nike says, "Just do it." There are a million or more excuses for not meditating, starting with "I don't have time" or "I'm too tired," but they are all simply excuses for not making your health a priority. No one has the time. How you spend your time is up to you.

Meditation has also been found to boost attention. In a study published in the *International Journal of Yoga*, researchers found that when children are trained to practice meditation, their attention spans are significantly increased. The researchers tested two yoga-based relaxation practices involving specific meditation and rest techniques with 208 school children (132 boys and 76 girls) between the ages of 13 and 16. Their attention spans were tested before and after practicing the meditation and rest techniques. Both techniques improved the children's attentiveness significantly, but meditation had the greatest impact on the attention scores, regardless of gender or age.[31]

While the study shows that meditation training may be valuable in improving attention in children and especially in the treatment of children with attention deficit hyperactivity disorder, it is likely that the effects translate to adults, as well.

How to Benefit

You can choose breathing meditation, walking meditation, sitting meditation, mindfulness meditation, guided meditation, visualization, or prayer. Most of these types of meditation indicate what is involved.

Commit to meditating for at least 10 minutes per day. Simply let go of thoughts that come to your mind. Don't try to force your thoughts to disappear. That doesn't usually work, anyway. Simply acknowledge thoughts and let them go. If your thoughts come back, acknowledge them again and let them go again, as often as needed. Meditation is like any other activity. Most of us need practice and patience to get the hang of it. And if you're just not disciplined enough to do it on your own, sign up for a local meditation group in your area. Many cities and towns have guided meditation groups to help people learn (and commit to) meditation on a regular basis.

Here is a simple, yet effective, meditation exercise. You can play peaceful background music while performing this meditation or you can have silence, whichever you prefer.

1. Sit in a comfortable position where you will not be disturbed. If you have children, it is important to teach them to respect your quiet time.

Taking time to recharge and release stress will allow you to be a better parent. Close your eyes. Keep your head upright and shoulders relaxed.

2. Begin by breathing deeply and steadily. Do not force your breathing. Simply breathe as deeply as you comfortably can. Observe your breath.

3. Begin to allow your breath to expand your abdomen. Comfortably expand your abdomen with each inhalation, and then release your abdomen with every exhalation.

4. Continue breathing deeply for at least 10 minutes. The longer you can meditate, the better.

Practice this meditation daily, increasing the amount of time each day. You can also purchase excellent guided meditation apps, CDs, videos, and DVDs to help with your meditation practice.[32]

Super Health Bonus

Research shows that meditation helps manage binge eating, emotional eating, and weight loss in overweight individuals who have these behaviors.[33] If you're overweight, you can expect that meditation will help address any tendencies toward emotional eating, such as binge eating or eating when you're stressed.

60-SECOND BRAIN HEALTH TIP #40:
Stretch and Cycle for a Superb Memory

Stretch your muscles and hop on a bike to boost both short-term and long-term memory.

Do you want to enhance your short- and long-term memory? Simply taking time out of your day to stretch your muscles and then hopping on your bike can significantly improve both types of memory.

Kirsten Hotting, PhD, of the University of Hamburg, in Germany, wanted to find out if exercise begun later in life could make a difference to memory. She evaluated 68 inactive women and men ages 40 to 56 and assigned them to either a stretching or a cycling program. An additional 18 inactive people acted as controls for the study. Each of the programs was supervised and lasted for 1 hour, twice weekly.

"The stretching/coordination training started with a short warmup phase, followed by stretching and strengthening of the major muscles of the whole body," Dr. Hotting said. "Coordination exercises were balance exercises, complex movements of arms and legs, and so on. The training ended with some relaxation exercises." The cyclists exercised at their target heart rate for 45 minutes and then finished with a cooldown pace. Her team measured memory and other cognitive skills.

The study found that those people who did stretching exercises for the same duration each week boosted their short-term memory, while the cyclists who rode for 1 or 2 hours weekly had a noticeable improvement in long-term memory after 6 months.[34] The study also suggests that mixing different types of exercises may have synergistic effects, boosting their overall brain benefits. Additionally, both the cycling and the stretching groups performed better on memory tests than the inactive group.

As you age, and particularly in late adulthood, your hippocampus—a part of your brain involved in memory—typically shrinks. Dr. Hotting's research shows that this part of your brain can actually grow after you begin to exercise. And that brain growth results in improved memory.

The cyclists performed better than both the stretching and inactive groups in long-term retention of learned material. The stretching group improved more in a test of attention than the cycling group. To test attention, the participants were given a paper and pencil test in which they had to find and mark certain letters quickly.

Earlier studies also found that inactive people who become physically active increase blood flow to the brain and score better on memory tests.[35]

How to Benefit

It's easier than you think to reap the memory benefits of stretching and exercise. Choose 2 days a week to perform stretching exercises for 1 hour each day. Choose an additional 2 days a week to cycle or perform another form of cardiovascular activity for at least 1 hour each day. (Keep in mind that the study participants cycled at their target heart rates for 45 minutes before engaging in a 15-minute cooldown.)

So how do you calculate your target heart rate? It's easier than you think. However, keep in mind that this is an estimate only and is primarily relevant to activities during which your feet touch the ground (such as walking or running). Women should subtract their age from 226 and men should subtract their age from 220. (For cycling, subtract 5 from your result to get your estimated maximum heart rate. For swimming, subtract 10 to get your estimated maximum heart rate.) Then multiply that top rate by 50 percent to get a minimum target heart rate and by 85 percent to get your maximum target heart rate. For example, a 40-year-old man would subtract 40 from 220 to get 180. Then he would multiply that amount by 0.50 to get 90, which is the low end of his target heart rate. He would then multiply 180 by 0.85 to get 153, which is his maximum target heart rate per minute.

Super Health Bonus

In the University of Hamburg study, the cyclist group improved their heart fitness by 15 percent, boosting their overall cardiovascular health. You can reap the same heart health benefits by participating in at least 1 hour of cycling twice a week.

60-SECOND BRAIN HEALTH TIP #41:
Game Your Way to a Supercharged Memory

Play games and puzzles to boost long- and short-term memory, information retention, and concentration.

The road to brain health may be more of a puzzling path—one filled with games and puzzles, that is. According to researchers at the University of California, Berkeley, any activity that stimulates the part of your brain that handles planning, memory, and abstract thinking offers a twofold benefit, strengthening both your brain and your immune system. That includes doing puzzles or playing games on a regular basis.

Other studies show that playing games can improve your short- and long-term memory, help you retain new information, and improve concentration. Even people who already suffer from a brain disease, including Alzheimer's disease, or a traumatic brain injury show mental improvement when they participate in memory games or computerized brain-training programs.

In a study published in the *Archives of Neurology*, researchers studied 10 people with Alzheimer's disease along with 65 healthy adults and 11 young people. They found that those who participated in mentally stimulating activities had less beta-amyloid—one of the suspected causes of Alzheimer's disease. The researchers concluded that people who participated in more brain games, reading, and writing in early and midlife have lower levels of beta-amyloid and a reduced likelihood of Alzheimer's disease.[36]

Additional research in the journal *Brain Injury* found that memory tests improved the memories of adult brain-injury patients. The study explored the effects of brain training on 21 adults who had suffered traumatic brain injuries an average of 37 months prior to the study. The participants conducted memory training on a computerized program on a daily basis for 5 weeks. Researchers assessed their results 4 weeks and 20 weeks after the memory training. The study's authors concluded that ". . . structured and intense computerized working memory training improves subjects' cognitive functioning."[37]

While you can benefit from participating in many different memory games, researched showed that participants in The Brain Fitness Program, a computerized brain-training program developed by Posit Science, experienced significant memory, attention, and information-processing improvements. The researchers found that participants scored as well on memory and attention as people 10 years younger who had not participated in the memory game.[38]

How to Benefit

For your convenience, my friends at *Prevention* magazine have singled out the 10 best brain-boosting games to improve your memory, retention, reaction time, concentration, and more—and they're fun, too! There's no need to sign up or pay a fee. Just visit prevention.com/content/brain-games to get started! You can choose to play two or three games a week, or you can play them all every day and challenge yourself to see how much you can improve throughout our program. Additionally, you can also dig out Scrabble or a jigsaw puzzle, or do the crossword or sudoku in your daily newspaper.

Super Health Bonus

Like I said, these games are fun, so they have the added bonus of helping to relieve stress, as well! And, as the University of California, Berkeley, scientists found, you'll be boosting your immune system at the same time. Catching fewer viruses isn't a bad side effect of having fun playing games or doing puzzles.

60-SECOND BRAIN HEALTH TIP #42:
Walk Your Way to a Bigger, Better Brain

A daily walk can stave off dementia.

You don't often think about taking your brain on a brisk walk or run, but that's the advice British researchers are offering after studying the potential ability of exercise to stave off dementia.[39]

Professor Clive Ballard researches age-related diseases at King's College London, and he has found that exercise has a more noticeable impact on slowing cognitive decline than completing puzzles, an activity that's proven to maintain brain health. (See 60-Second Brain Health Tip #41 on page 150.) Specifically, brisk walking or moderate jogging for 40 minutes three times a week will help people protect themselves from the ravages of dementia.

Dr. Ballard's work echoes findings from the University of Pittsburgh. Researchers at the university found that participants in their study experienced brain growth after three weekly sessions of moderate exercise, such as a fast-paced 40-minute walk. Considering your brain shrinks by about 1 percent annually, the researchers considered a 2 percent increase in brain size to be significant. They also found that exercise participants between the ages of 55 and 80 experienced an increase in the size of the hippocampus, the part of the brain largely responsible for memory and our ability to discern spatial relationships.

Research by the University of Cambridge and the National Institute on Aging explored the exercise–brain health connection in mice. Scientists found that mice that ran an average of 15 miles a day doubled the memory test scores of their sedentary companions.[40] Fortunately, humans don't have to run mini-marathons to reap the benefits of taking their brains out for some exercise.

Dr. Ballard, who is leading a long-term study on "brain training" for older people, found that intellectual games such as crossword puzzles offer little positive impact on brain health when it comes to cognitive disorders that fall under the general term of dementia. He also found that they did not offer protection against Alzheimer's disease, arguably the most well-known form of dementia. That's not a reason to stop enjoying your crosswords and sudoku puzzles. Just remember to regularly get up off the couch and take your brain for a lap around the block.

We all know that we need to get moving, but additional research gives us one more reason to stay or become active. According to a large review published in the *BMJ*, researchers from Harvard University, Stanford University, and Britain's London School of Economics and Political Science assessed 305 studies of 340,000 people and found that exercise was more effective than prescription drugs for stroke recovery. As an interesting aside, they also found no statistical differences between the effects of exercise or drugs for people suffering from heart disease or prediabetic symptoms.

Considering the high cost of many prescription drugs and the potentially serious health risks, exercise is a superior choice. It has also been shown to reduce your risk of depression. However, I'm not suggesting that you stop taking any drugs that your doctor may have prescribed, just that you add a reasonable amount of physical activity to your day.

And considering that the World Health Organization indicates that physical inactivity is the fourth leading risk factor for death, causing approximately 3.2 million deaths worldwide every year, there's more reason than ever to get started.

The researchers at Harvard, Stanford, and London's School of Economics recommended that doctors write prescriptions for exercise, which seems to be having an effect in communities like Leduc, Alberta, Canada.[41] Doctors in this community recognized the power of the prescription pad and put it to work to get the community in shape. For a year, doctors handed out "Prescriptions to Get Active," with information regarding the specific exercise type, intensity, and duration for each patient. Over 200 patients followed the doctors' advice. According to Justin Balko, MD, president of the Leduc Beaumont Devon Primary Care Network, he was inspired by research he read in New Zealand medical journals that showed prescriptions for exercise increased physical activity in adults by 10 percent for at least a year in that country. But you don't need a prescription to reap the brain benefits of exercise. In another study in the journal *Brain Sciences*, scientists found that even a few months of physical exercise increased cognition and improved brain functions in previously sedentary adults. The study participants ranged in age from 42 to 57 years old.[42] The scientists found a direct link between verbal learning and memory and cardiovascular fitness. You achieve that by doing the kind of exercise that gets your heart pumping. So lace up your walking shoes, hit the streets, swing those arms, and watch your brain health improve.

How to Benefit

You don't need any expensive equipment or designer gear to benefit from the research that links walking and exercise to a healthier brain and a reduced risk of brain diseases such as depression. All you have to do is motivate yourself to get moving every day. If you find it easier at a certain time of day, then stick to that time every day, at least 5 days a week. You could walk home from work instead of driving. Or you could take the stairs instead of an elevator. Or before you crash in front of the television after dinner, head outside for a walk. There's no wrong way. Just do whatever works best for you.

Super Health Bonus

You won't just boost brain health; you'll boost your lung and heart health, as well. By breathing deeper and getting your blood pumping harder, you'll be oxygenating your blood, which improves oxygen flow to every cell and tissue in your body.

Many studies show that regular exercise reduces your risk of colon and breast cancer, bone fractures, obesity, diabetes, and cardiovascular diseases. While you're busy sending oxygen-rich blood to your brain to help it function better, you'll also reduce your risk of many other health conditions.

60-SECOND BRAIN HEALTH TIP #43:

Practice Mind over Platter Because Portion Size Matters

Kick the overeating habit to significantly reduce memory loss and cognitive impairment.

You've already learned which foods and ingredients to avoid, as well as which ones are the best brain foods, but when it comes to eating for a healthy brain, there is more to the equation.

New research shows that overeating may double your risk of memory loss. The study, published by the American Academy of Neurology, found that the more calories eaten each day, the higher a person's risk of developing mental impairment at age 70 and above. Researchers studied 1,200 people between the ages of 70 and 79, including individuals with and without mild cognitive impairment. Mild cognitive impairment is defined as the stage between age-related memory loss and full-blown Alzheimer's disease. The study participants were divided into three groups based on the number of calories eaten each day. Scientists concluded that the group of people who ate the most calories daily had twice the risk of experiencing mild cognitive impairment.[43]

It seems that habitual overeating causes memory loss and cognitive impairment. Based on the study results, we also know that avoiding overeating and eating a healthy, brain-boosting diet like the one described throughout *60 Seconds to Boost Your Brain Power* can protect your brain from significant memory loss.

How to Benefit

Cutting calories and eating healthy does more than preserve your physical health—it also protects your brain from significant memory loss. Looked at another way, habitual overeating appears to directly *cause* memory loss and cognitive impairment. So how do you eat less without going hungry? Let's explore an interesting study examining people's eating habits and the psychology behind overeating.

You know you should stop eating that pile of food on your plate, but it's soooo good and it's just so hard to stop. How much will you eat? According to a new study titled "Mind over Platter" and conducted at the University of Bristol's School of Experimental Psychology in the United Kingdom, several things affect how much food we eat,[44] including:

Portion size. The more food you pile up on your plate, the more food you'll eat. According to research cited in the *Atlantic*, on average, we eat about 92 percent of all the food on our plates, regardless of how much food we pile on.[45] So if we hit the buffet and stack our food sky-high, we'll probably eat 92 percent of it; conversely, if we stick to a small plate of "rabbit food," we're still likely to eat 92 percent of it. This is a serious concern in North America, where portion sizes at many restaurants, fast-food joints, and even at home have grown alongside our collective waistbands. As portion sizes grow, so will our risk of cognitive impairment, as well as our likelihood of obesity, if we keep eating 92 percent of everything in front of us. Knowing this means that you should cut back on the amount you pile on your plate.

Whether the food is "bottomless." When people eat from a self-refilling soup bowl, people keep on eating. Meal size grows, even though people do not report feeling more full than when they eat less. When you're in a restaurant, skip the buffets and other meal options that replenish what you've eaten.

How well we remember our last meal. When people are reminded of another meal they ate, they slow down on consumption of their current meal. In other words, when someone reminds us of the big lunch we ate, we tend to eat less at dinner. There's no big surprise there, but it makes me wonder whether the results are because we feel guilty that we shouldn't eat so much or if simply remembering a recent meal tends to make us feel fuller. Either way, take a quick minute before a meal to remind yourself of how much food you've eaten in a day.

Whether we have company. While most people may think they eat more while watching television, research showed that we eat more when we are alone and there is nothing to distract us from our food. Undistracted and on our own, we eat 97 percent of the food on our plates, but if we eat with others or with the TV on, we eat 89 percent of our food. As much as possible, eat with friends or family members. And don't feel so bad for those times you drop in front of the television to enjoy your dinner.

Super Health Bonus

Not only will cutting back on your caloric intake reduce your risk of cognitive decline and the size of your waistline, extensive research shows that doing so on a regular basis may actually increase longevity. So you may find that you live longer when you make a small effort to eat a bit less each day.

Brain Books in Action

NAME: Shelagh Pritchard

AGE: 58

OCCUPATION: Director of an NGO

"I've learned that if you don't eat perfectly every day, it doesn't mean you are failing at the task you've set for yourself. What it does mean is that you love yourself enough to keep trying and learning how to improve."

How I Got Here: After Shelagh Pritchard's father began to experience memory issues following a major heart attack, she started to look closely at the health patterns in her family and the potential impact on her own life. Shelagh learned that dementia is often linked to lifestyle issues and genetic factors, so she quickly decided to be proactive versus reactive in addressing any problems lurking in her own future. When Shelagh was invited to be a part of a test panel for this book, even though she had not experienced any memory or health problems of her own, she jumped at the opportunity to see how some simple changes might make a difference in her brain health and her everyday life.

Progress Report: Unfortunately, when the 4-week test panel began, another member of Shelagh's family experienced a serious health emergency, so she spent the first 3 weeks away from home and in caretaker mode, trying to finesse the eating plan while being unable to cook for herself in her own kitchen. "I found it difficult to focus on the task and plan ahead for my meals. And the emotional stress I was under made me want to eat comfort foods instead of making healthier choices."

Because Shelagh was on the road so much and attending to her family member and related hospital visits, she found it easiest to start with the exercises and strategies outlined in *60 Seconds to Boost Your Brain Power* and to introduce the food plan afterward. She also spent time carefully reviewing the program, making notes on information that was new to her and keeping a list of supplements and foods to add to her diet. Looking back, Shelagh points out that the simple practice of paying attention to these details made it easier for her to remain mindful of better food choices and track how she felt after eating certain foods.

Beyond: Shelagh continues to practice mindfulness when it comes to her food choices. "I notice that for me better nutrition means I have more energy and quicker thinking," she explains. "Every day is not perfect, but I see small improvements, so I am encouraged to continue."

CHAPTER 6

WEEK 4: SUPPLEMENT

Use These Supplements to Supercharge Your Brain Health and Memory

This week you'll learn about the best brain-boosting nutrients, herbs, and medicinal mushrooms that can help you prevent brain diseases, boost your memory, or treat specific brain conditions. As you'll soon see, many of these natural supplements have been proven both safe and effective. While you may have learned about some of the foods that contain these brain-building substances in Chapter 4, supplements can often provide a much higher dose of the active ingredients than foods alone offer. You should choose at least two of the supplements from this chapter, but of course, you can choose more if you want to. Read through each tip to learn about the strengths of each supplement to find the ones that best fit your health needs. Simply place a check beside each of the supplements you've selected to help you stay on track.

In this section, you'll learn to:

44. Give Your Gut a Boost for Better Brain Health (page 162)

Certain strains of probiotics have proven brain health benefits and even help prevent brain diseases.

45. Boost Your Brain Protection with B Vitamins (page 165)

B-complex vitamins like niacin, folate, and B$_{12}$ are essential nutrients for a healthy brain and for the formation of brain messengers known as neurotransmitters.

46. Combine Forces with CoQ10 to Create Brain Energy (page 170)

Give your brain cells an energy boost with the natural nutrient coenzyme Q10.

47. Enhance Your Levels of Vitamin E to Protect Brain Cells (page 172)

Research shows that vitamin E is more effective in the treatment of Alzheimer's disease than any pharmaceutical drug on the market.

48. Give Your Brain Chemicals a Boost with the Nutrient 5-HTP (page 173)

Boost your mood and prevent mood swings with the "happy hormone."

49. Go for Gold with Ginkgo (page 175)

Ginkgo helps slow the effects of aging, reduces your risk of dementia, and is a proven medical treatment for Alzheimer's disease.

50. Make Magnesium Your Go-To Mineral (page 178)

Low magnesium levels, a common occurrence, are linked to decreased cognitive function.

51. Pick Periwinkle: The Blue Flower for Gray Matter (page 180)

Boost your short-term memory or treat dementia with this potent blue flower.

52. Recycle Brain-Healing Nutrients with Alpha Lipoic Acid (page 182)

This powerful nutrient protects both the watery and the fatty parts of your brain from free radical damage.

53. Seek a Wise Sage (page 185)

Boost your mood and short- and long-term memory with sage oil.

54. Sniff Lavender for a Mood Boost (page 187)

Conquer depression with the flower that has proven itself more effective than antidepressant drugs.

55. Pick Curcumin for a Better Brain (page 189)

Give your brain a significant memory boost within an hour of taking this potent nutrient.

56. Seize Fish Oil Supplements for Superior Intellect (page 192)

Give yourself a bigger, more resilient brain with fish oil supplements.

57. Gain New Hope for Parkinson's Disease with Gastrodin (page 193)

This natural supplement, derived from Chinese orchids, treats headaches, stroke, and even Parkinson's disease.

58. Select Cordyceps to Prevent and Treat Stroke (page 195)

Prevent and treat stroke with the medicinal mushroom proven to boost learning and memory, too.

59. Race for Brilliance with Reishi Mushrooms (page 197)

Protect your brain from seizures, Huntington's disease, and stroke damage with this amazing medicinal mushroom.

60-SECOND BRAIN HEALTH TIP #44:
Give Your Gut a Boost for Better Brain Health

Certain strains of probiotics have proven brain health benefits and even help prevent brain diseases.

When we think of brain diseases, Alzheimer's disease, dementia, Lou Gehrig's disease, and Parkinson's disease come to mind. While the treatments for these conditions tend to be complex and ideally involve many brain-boosting foods and natural medicines, new research suggests that probiotics have a place in the prevention and treatment of these brain conditions, as well.

That's because cutting-edge research shows that probiotics can function as antioxidants in your body, reducing the effects of aging. This is especially good news for sufferers of brain diseases and those who wish to prevent them. Your brain is particularly vulnerable to free radical damage, especially the 60 percent of your brain that is made up of fat. Probiotics help to protect the fatty parts of your brain from damage and this, in turn, helps prevent brain diseases like those mentioned above.

The research into using probiotics for brain health is still fairly new, but the promise and wide-reaching implications it holds are exciting, particularly because the incidence of brain disease is on the rise.

"What happens in Vegas stays in Vegas," but the same can't be said of your gut. What happens in your gut plays a role in determining the health of your brain. These seemingly unrelated parts of your body are actually intimately connected. When it comes to your health, it is more accurately stated as "What happens in your bowels determines the health of your brain." Sounds crazy, but it's true. Here are two reasons why your digestive health plays an enormous role in your brain health.

1. You've likely heard that "You are what you eat." But I think "You are what you eat, digest, absorb, and assimilate" is a better way to put it. After all, what you eat, digest, absorb, and assimilate will become the

building blocks of every cell in your body, including those in your brain. If your digestion processes are impaired, your body will lack adequate building blocks to maintain healthy brain and nervous system cells.

2. Research is showing that the gastrointestinal tract plays a huge part in your body's immune response. It is one of the main determinants of the levels of inflammation in your body and whether your body will attack healthy tissue. And you may recall our discussion about the inflammation–brain connection in Chapter 1. Getting on top of inflammation is critical to maintaining healthy brain function.

So how do you boost your gut health to build a healthier brain? First let's explore some essentials of gut health: Over 100,000,000,000,000 (that's 100 trillion!) bacteria of more than 400 different species reside in your intestines. Actually, there are more microorganisms found in your digestive tract than there are cells in your body. Most of these bacteria live in your large intestine, which is also known as the colon. You may be alarmed at the very thought of bacteria living in your body, but these bacteria are an important part of your health. They help ensure that food is adequately broken down, nutrients are synthesized and absorbed, toxins are eliminated so they cannot be absorbed into your blood, harmful bacteria stay in check, and your immune system is healthy. These beneficial bacteria are also known as flora, microflora, or probiotics (the opposite of antibiotics, which kill bacteria indiscriminately).

The two main types of beneficial bacteria, which are also called "friendly bacteria," are *Lactobacilli* and *Bifidobacteria*. Research is beginning to show that these two types of microflora can lower your body's levels of toxic compounds that could have detrimental effects on your brain.

Studies show that these bacteria lower immune system compounds called cytokines in your gut, and also throughout your bloodstream. Cytokines are linked to anxiety, symptoms of depression, and cognitive disturbances in healthy adults. Cytokines also lower levels of an important brain and nerve cell protector.

Lactobacilli and *Bifidobacteria* act as antioxidants in your body. Multiple studies demonstrate probiotics' protective ability against free radical damage, especially against damage to the fatty component of cells. Your brain is largely made of fat, so protecting the fatty component of cells from free radical damage is important to brain health. Here are two of the studies.

One study by Dr. Tatyana Oxman and her Israeli colleagues showed that *L. bulgaricus* protected heart cells against the effects of insufficient oxygenated blood. In the same study, the group of people taking this strain of *L. bulgaricus* also had a 42 percent reduction in a particular type of inflammatory cytokines.

Research conducted at UCLA and published in the *American Journal of Clinical Nutrition* found that consuming certain probiotics could actually produce many brain health benefits, including some linked to sensory and emotional processing. Swedish researchers found that *L. plantarum* resulted in a 37 percent reduction in the chemicals linked to free radical damage that are elevated in many brain and nerve disorders. They originally studied the effects of these bacteria on smokers to see if probiotics had any protective effects.[1] Free radical damage has been linked to brain and nerve diseases, making their research particularly important for those suffering from brain diseases. The researchers also observed the effects of particular inflammatory compounds called interleukin-6 (IL-6). These compounds are elevated in brain diseases, so reducing them through the use of probiotics is helpful in the treatment of brain diseases.[2]

The use of probiotics as a potential treatment for brain diseases is still in its infancy, but considering their lack of side effects, affordability, and availability, as well as the many other health benefits that come with using them, it is a natural fit within a larger treatment plan for brain diseases.

How to Benefit

Ideally, take them with some water on an empty stomach. Choose a high-quality product that contains a range of proven strains in the *Lactobacillus* and *Bifidobacteria* families. You'll notice that these names are frequently shortened on product labels to *L.* and *B.*, respectively. Look for *L. acidophilus, L. bifidus, L. bulgaricus,* and *L. plantarum*, since the former two are proven gut-health builders and the latter two have been shown in studies to boost brain health. Other beneficial strains include *L. rhamnosus, Bifidobacterium bifidum, B. longum,* and *B. subtilis.* While it is important to take a high-potency product, it is not merely a numbers game. In other words, sometimes products with claims of many billion colony-forming units, the measure of how many probiotics of a particular strain are found in the product, don't contain the numbers they claim to. For more information about selecting a good probiotic, consult my book *The Probiotic Promise*. You can also check out my Web site at DrMichelleCook.com to learn about specific products I recommend.

Super Health Bonus

When you supplement with probiotics, you can expect to experience improved digestion and reduced gut inflammation. That's because probiotics have been proven in many studies to have beneficial effects on digestion and to have an anti-inflammatory effect. Research at Osaka University School of Medicine found that certain strains of probiotics even reduce allergy symptoms.[3] So you may even notice fewer allergy symptoms if you are an allergy sufferer.

60-SECOND BRAIN HEALTH TIP #45:
Boost Your Brain Protection with B Vitamins

B-complex vitamins like niacin, folate, and B_{12} are essential nutrients for a healthy brain and the formation of brain messengers known as neurotransmitters.

Every cell in your body needs particular vitamins to work properly, and your brain is no different. Without adequate B-complex vitamins, cellular functions begin to break down until there are potentially serious flaws in their workings. If this happens, the cells may even die off prematurely as your body tries to protect itself against possible damage, which is called apoptosis. The main B-complex vitamins required by brain cells include niacin (B_3), folate (B_9), and B_{12}.

All B vitamins are important for the formation of neurotransmitters, the hormones that act as messengers in your brain. These hormones help regulate your brain's many functions, including healthy mood balance. Most people have some deficiencies of the B-complex vitamins, especially B_{12}, which tends to be more difficult to absorb with age.

Your brain tends to shrink with age. Scientists have been studying why this happens, and more importantly, what can slow brain shrinkage. They found that B vitamins may hold at least part of the solution. One study followed 168 people who, for 2 years, were given either a placebo that contained no B vitamins or a B vitamin supplement containing high doses of folic acid, vitamin C, and vitamin B_{12}. Researchers found that the brains of people taking the vitamin supplement had brain shrinkage at a rate of 0.76 percent per year, while those taking the placebo had an average brain shrinkage rate of 1.08 percent, which is a significant difference.[4] A small amount of brain shrinkage over many years may be normal, but not at the rates people are currently experiencing. And Alzheimer's disease, Parkinson's disease, and other brain diseases are not normal parts of aging, either. By making simple dietary and lifestyle changes, as well as supplement additions, we can drastically cut the risk of experiencing any of these conditions. B-complex vitamins are great brain health support.

Since B-complex vitamins work best when combined, they are often sold in combination form in tablets or capsules. However, if you are already suffering from a brain disorder, you may need specific individual B vitamins, as well. In that case, it is still best to take a B-complex vitamin and add extra B_{12} or folic acid, for example.

Niacin (vitamin B_3). Niacin protects against Alzheimer's disease, suggests a study published in the *Journal of Neurology, Neurosurgery, and Psychiatry*.[5] It appears to protect your brain by stimulating the production of acetylcholine, which can be destroyed by organophosphates. Niacin is critical for proper activity of the brain chemical acetylcholine.[6] Dementia can even be caused by a severe deficiency of niacin, which ongoing supplementation with niacin can resolve.[7]

Folate (vitamin B$_9$). Low levels of the B vitamin folate have been linked to an increased risk of developing Alzheimer's disease or depression. Folate protects nerves and brain cells from damage. Conversely, research shows that supplementation with folate helps to reverse or slow cognitive decline. That's likely because folate helps protect nerve and brain cells from damage. Low folate levels increase your risk of developing Alzheimer's disease.[8]

Low levels of folate have also been linked to depression. Research presented at the Alzheimer's Association meeting in Washington, DC, showed that a high dose (800 micrograms [mcg]) of folic acid daily may slow cognitive decline related to aging. This amount is equivalent to 2½ pounds of strawberries. Researchers tested more than 800 people with good cognitive functioning for 3 years. Those who were given the supplement scored 5.5 years younger than their age. On tests for cognitive speed, they scored as well as people 1.9 years younger.

Additional research from the Human Nutrition Research Center on Aging at Tufts University in Boston assessed folate levels in an ethnically diverse group of 2,948 people between 15 and 39 years old. Three hundred and one individuals in the group were diagnosed with major depression and 121 were diagnosed with dysthymia (a chronically depressed mood present more than 50 percent of the time for at least 2 years). Researchers found that people who were diagnosed with major depression had lower red blood cell and serum folate concentrations than people who had never been diagnosed with depression. People with dysthymia also had lower red blood cell and folate levels than people who had never been diagnosed with the disease. Their research suggests a correlation between a folate deficiency and depressive disorders. It's fair to conclude that supplementing with folate may be a beneficial treatment for depressive disorders and that maintaining sufficient levels of folate may help prevent depression.[9]

Vitamin B_{12}. All B vitamins help brain cells communicate with each other by assisting with the production of brain hormones called neurotransmitters. B_{12} is especially important because it helps your body produce the neurotransmitter acetylcholine, which allows nerve cells to transmit memory signals. Studies even link a B_{12} deficiency to an increased risk of Alzheimer's disease or Alzheimer's-like symptoms of memory loss.[10] A study in the journal *Clinical Therapeutics* showed that memory-related symptoms diminished when people received injections of vitamin B_{12}.[11] (Of course, most people don't need B_{12} injections and can simply take over-the-counter supplements. See page 169 for more information.) B_{12} deficiencies have also been linked to depression, and supplementation with the nutrient has shown promise in the treatment of depression.[12] Research has also shown that low levels of vitamin B_{12} are linked with poorer memory function in older people with a high risk for Alzheimer's.[13] Among healthy people over the age of 75 who have a genetic predisposition associated with increased risk for Alzheimer's, low levels of vitamin B_{12} are associated with significantly worse performance on memory tests, according to a study published in *Neuropsychology*.[14]

In numerous studies, B vitamins, particularly B_6, B_{12}, niacin, and folate, demonstrated the ability to lower levels of an artery-hardening chemical called homocysteine, which is found in the blood and linked to stroke. Excess homocysteine can also lead to memory disorders and Alzheimer's disease, according to a study in the *Journal of Nutrition, Health & Aging*.[15] If you're asking "To B or not to B (supplement, that is)?" I'm definitely in favor of "to B."

How to Benefit

While it is always a good idea to obtain B vitamins from foods such as eggs, fish, legumes, gluten-free whole grains, and nuts, it is wise to take a B-complex supplement, as well. Alternatively, be sure that your high-quality multivitamin contains adequate B vitamins. Most people will benefit from supplementation with 50 milligrams (mg) of most of the B-complex vitamins, with the exception of

micrograms, not milligrams. In these
milligrams of other B vitamins will also
ate and B₁₂.

research above, you may feel inclined
f so, be sure to take a B-complex supple-
vitamins are a good fit for you. If you're
mmend that you work with a qualified
d in orthomolecular medicine (the use
us health conditions).

If you're adding niacin, you may wish to use niacinamide, because higher doses of niacin can cause a hot, flushing experience known as a "niacin flush." Niacinamide does not cause this effect. Taking 500 mg twice a day may help with dementia. Higher doses may be necessary, but again, it is best to work with an orthomolecular medicine practitioner in such cases.

Along with a B-complex supplement, 800 mcg of additional folate may be beneficial. The typically recommended dosage is 400 mcg daily.

Take 1,000 mcg of B_{12} for the prevention of or as part of a treatment plan for brain disorders. As we age, however, stomach acid typically declines, so it is beneficial to take extra vitamin B_{12}. An additional 1,000 mcg is beneficial if you have low stomach acid, are over 50, or are suffering from any brain disorder. Some people have low levels of a substance called intrinsic factor, which is normally found in the stomach. Intrinsic factor helps with the absorption of B_{12}. If you don't produce adequate intrinsic factor (and the only way to find out is through medical tests), you may benefit from vitamin B_{12} injections. If you have memory problems and are taking B_{12} nutritional supplements, you may want to get your doctor to test for an intrinsic-factor deficiency.

Super Health Bonus

B-complex vitamins, such as niacin, folate, and B_{12}, can boost your energy levels and reduce the harmful substance known as homocysteine, which is linked to premature aging and conditions such as heart disease.

60-SECOND BRAIN HEALTH TIP #46:

Combine Forces with CoQ10 to Create Brain Energy

Give your brain cells an energy boost with the natural nutrient coenzyme Q10.

In research, the nutrient coenzyme Q10 (or CoQ10, for short) has been shown to slow the progression of brain diseases, including Parkinson's. In other research, it has been shown to boost the energy centers in brain cells, thereby improving mental functioning and mood. It is a brain rejuvenator even for healthy people with no signs of brain disease.

CoQ10, which is needed to provide energy to your cells, is a naturally occurring substance found in your body and in some foods. Inside your cells there are micro-size energy-manufacturing facilities known as the mitochondria. Mitochondria depend on CoQ10 to boost energy for every cellular function, including brain functions. Unfortunately, this nutrient can become depleted as we age or experience health issues that require additional amounts, as in the case of brain diseases.

A study presented at the annual meeting of the American Neurological Association in New York City suggests that the nutritional supplement CoQ10 could slow the progression of Parkinson's disease. Lead researcher Professor Clifford Shults of the University of California, San Diego, and his colleagues enrolled 80 early-stage, non-levodopa-taking Parkinson's patients for the trial. (Levodopa is one of the main drugs used to treat Parkinson's disease.) The patients were randomly assigned treatment with 300, 600, or 1,200 mg per day of the nutrient CoQ10 or a placebo. After 8 months, patients who received the highest dose of CoQ10 fared significantly better than those who received the placebo. These highest-dose patients had a 44 percent reduction in disease progression, compared to the placebo group. Even patients taking only 300 mg per day of CoQ10 were better able to carry out simple daily activities, such as dressing and washing, and demonstrated better mental functioning and mood. Shults stresses that his study was small and therefore inconclusive;

however, it suggests that CoQ10 may slow the progression of neurodegenerative diseases, including Parkinson's.[16]

Earlier research provides evidence that the mitochondria, also known as the powerhouses of the body's cells, are impaired in Parkinson's patients.[17] Research also shows that CoQ10 is essential for proper energy production by these powerhouses.

Parkinson's is not the only brain disease that might benefit from CoQ10 supplementation. Alzheimer's has been linked to mutations in the mitochondria of the DNA. Researchers found variations of a specific DNA mutation in the brains of 65 percent of people with Alzheimer's disease and none in those without the disease.[18] While it is unclear whether the mutation is a contributing cause or an effect of the disease, attempting to ensure healthy, functioning mitochondria is essential to great brain health, and CoQ10 plays an important role.

Even if you're not suffering from any brain disease and simply want to give your brain all the fuel it needs to stay healthy, CoQ10 is worth serious consideration because it helps maintain healthy brain functions by providing brain cells with the energy they need. Plus, most people I've worked with report higher physical energy levels while taking CoQ10. I've been taking this supplement daily for close to 2 decades and can definitely say that it gives me an energy boost and helps keep brain fog at bay.

How to Benefit

CoQ10 is available in both supplement and lozenge form. If you're healthy and looking for additional brain health protection, take 100 mg daily. If you're suffering from a brain disease such as Alzheimer's or Parkinson's, you may need a higher dose, such as 300 mg. If your health issues are severe, you may wish to take an even higher dose than that. Professor Shults's study explored doses as high as 1,200 mg. Because CoQ10 is a naturally occurring substance in your body, it is fairly safe to use. There are no reported side effects of high doses. If you select CoQ10 lozenges, make sure the amount of sweetener they contain is extremely low (less than a few grams) and that they're devoid of preservatives and colors. If you're going to take higher amounts of CoQ10 daily, choose the supplement form, as the sugar from taking so many lozenges will be excessive.

Super Health Bonus

CoQ10 helps energize all of your body's functions and even gives a physical boost of energy, so don't be surprised if you feel less fatigued and more energetic throughout the day while supplementing with it.

60-SECOND BRAIN HEALTH TIP #47:
Enhance Your Levels of Vitamin E to Protect Brain Cells

Research shows that vitamin E is more effective in the treatment of Alzheimer's disease than any pharmaceutical drug on the market.

Vitamin E offers antioxidant protection to the fatty portion of your brain while reducing inflammation and your risk of brain damage. Powerful antioxidants such as vitamin E fight excess free radical damage that can interfere with how brain cells function. Over time, too many free radicals wear out brain cells and prevent them from communicating properly with each other, which can lead to memory loss.

The *New England Journal of Medicine* reported that vitamin E is more effective in treating Alzheimer's disease than any pharmaceutical drug on the market.[19] Another study reported in the *Journal of the American Geriatrics Society* found that inadequate antioxidant intake may increase a person's risk of cognitive decline.[20] Antioxidants such as vitamin E are also showing promise in their ability to protect your brain from damage. Additional research found that diets rich in vitamin E–containing foods were associated with a reduced risk of Alzheimer's disease.[21]

Vitamin E is the best-researched antioxidant for its supportive role in maintaining brain and memory function. The *Archives of Neurology* reported that in a group of 2,889 adults over age 65, those who had the highest vitamin E intake had the lowest rate of cognitive decline.[22] Another study in the *New England Journal of Medicine* showed that people with moderately severe Alzheimer's disease who supplemented with 2,000 international units (IU) per day of vitamin E slowed the disease's progression.[23] Other studies found that people with Alzheimer's or dementia have low levels of vitamins C and E, both of which are antioxidants your body uses to destroy free radicals.

How to Benefit

While it is imperative to eat foods rich in antioxidants because they are better used by your body than supplements, it is also important to supplement with additional vitamin E to protect your brain against damaging free radicals. Foods that are high in vitamin E include whole grains, almonds, sunflower seeds, and avocados. Supplement with 400 IU of vitamin E daily. Avoid taking larger doses unless you are working with a naturally minded health practitioner who is well versed in therapeutic doses of vitamin E. The vitamin can be stored in your body, and excess amounts can build up if large doses are taken.

Super Health Bonus

Vitamin E supplementation also boosts skin health and helps keep skin soft and supple.

60-SECOND BRAIN HEALTH TIP #48:

Give Your Brain Chemicals a Boost with the Nutrient 5-HTP

Boost your mood and prevent mood swings with the "happy hormone."
      Low levels of the nutrient 5-HTP have been linked with depression and mood regulation disorders. That's because 5-HTP is a precursor to the brain

hormone serotonin, which is known as the "happy hormone" due to its mood-balancing and elevating qualities. Serotonin is one of the brain neurotransmitters that allow brain cells to communicate.

Low levels of serotonin are frequently seen in people suffering from depression. Additionally, research shows that Parkinson's patients may have low levels of serotonin before they start to experience the motor symptoms characteristic of the disease, leading researchers to believe that, in some cases, depression may be one of the earliest symptoms of Parkinson's disease.[24]

The nutrient name 5-HTP stands for 5-hydroxytryptophan. It is usually derived from a naturally occurring substance from the seedpods of a West African medicinal plant known as *Griffonia simplicifolia*. In your body, 5-HTP is one of the raw materials needed to manufacture adequate serotonin levels. The success of 5-HTP in treating conditions like depression and mood imbalances that are linked to low serotonin levels has been extensively documented.

While you can't take a serotonin pill to boost your levels, you can help your body manufacture more of it by supplementing with 5-HTP. (The herb St. John's wort can also help with boosting serotonin levels and in the treatment of mild to moderate depression.)

The effectiveness of treating depression with 5-HTP supplements has been known for many years. As early as the 1980s, research in the journals *Advances in Biochemical Psychopharmacology* and *Biological Psychiatry* found that taking a 5-HTP supplement could be valuable in the treatment of depression.[25, 26]

How to Benefit

If you're not suffering from mood imbalances or depression, you probably don't need 5-HTP. The supplement is best reserved for the treatment of depression or depression linked to Parkinson's disease. In both cases, it is best to work with a qualified nutritionist and/or a physician who is knowledgeable about natural medicine (unfortunately, most aren't) and who can monitor your serotonin levels and adjust your dose of 5-HTP as necessary. The standard dose for depression is 50 mg three times daily. If symptoms have not improved after 2 weeks, increase the dosage to 100 mg three times daily. Occasionally, nausea is a side effect of taking 5-HTP, but gradually increasing the dose in this manner helps to lessen the possibility of nausea. Enteric-coated capsules or tablets are also helpful, and you can take the supplement with food. As with all supplements, be sure to choose a reputable brand, because there are major variations in quality and active ingredient content between different manufacturers. For more information on supplement brands, visit my Web site at DrMichelleCook.com.

Super Health Bonus

Supplementation with 5-HTP has been found to be beneficial to insomniacs.[27] So if you're suffering from insomnia, you may find that 5-HTP helps. Additionally, other research shows that it may help reduce symptoms of fibromyalgia.[28]

60-SECOND BRAIN HEALTH TIP #49:
Go for Gold with Ginkgo

Ginkgo helps slow the effects of aging, reduces your risk of dementia, and is a proven medical treatment for Alzheimer's disease.

The ginkgo biloba tree you see today is almost identical to the one that stood alongside dinosaurs during the Jurassic period. The ginkgo tree is perhaps one of the oldest trees on the planet, reaching over 100 feet tall when fully mature and even surviving the Ice Age.

Ginkgo biloba has been extensively used for millennia to improve blood flow to the brain and to relieve dementia, depression, vertigo, tinnitus, multiple sclerosis, nerve pain, and fragile blood vessels.[29] Even the *Journal of the American Medical Association,* which has traditionally been quite conservative in offering claims about natural medicines, has acknowledged that ginkgo might help slow the effects of old age on the brain (which they refer to as senile dementia).[30]

In Germany, the herb ginkgo biloba is even approved as a medical treatment for Alzheimer's disease. Ginkgo has a long history of use among natural health practitioners and herbalists to boost memory function and support brain health against illnesses such as depression and stroke. Ginkgo appears to work by increasing the oxygen supply to your brain and the availability of energy to brain cells.

In a study of 40 patients with early-stage Alzheimer's disease, researchers found that 240 mg of ginkgo biloba extract taken daily for 3 months produced noticeable improvements in memory, mood, and attention.[31] Hundreds of European studies have demonstrated ginkgo's proven ability to help with a wide variety of conditions linked to aging, including memory loss and poor circulation.[32]

While ginkgo is beneficial for treating brain diseases, it is also an excellent preventive medicine. That's because one of the main ways ginkgo works is by improving circulation, both in your brain and throughout your body.

There are two main types of active ingredients in ginkgo: flavonoids and terpenes. Flavonoids are powerful antioxidants that neutralize damaging free radicals in your brain and body before they can do damage. Because free radicals are chemically imbalanced molecules, they bind to healthy cells, damaging them in the process. Free radicals in the brain are linked to impaired memory and brain damage, so getting and keeping them under control is one of the keys to a healthy brain. Fortunately, ginkgo is a rich source of free radical–quelling flavonoids.

There are terpenes found in ginkgo that are not found in other substances, including bilobalides and ginkgolides. These terpenes are antioxidants that improve circulation and protect your brain against damage, but they have also been found to improve memory and mental function and to aid in stroke recovery.[33]

According to Commission E, Germany's official panel of doctors, pharmacologists, and experts who review herbal medicines for safety and effectiveness, ginkgo has many other effects. This herb:

- Increases your body's tolerance of lack of oxygen, especially in brain tissue
- Inhibits swelling in the brain caused by trauma or toxins
- Reduces swelling and lesions in the retinas
- Inhibits an age-related decline of choline receptors (choline is an important nutrient found in brain and nerve tissue) and promotes choline uptake in your brain
- Improves memory and learning capacity
- Helps improve balance
- Improves blood flow, especially in the capillaries
- Scavenges free radicals
- Inhibits the platelet activating factor, a mediator of chemical processes within your body, including platelet aggregation, blood clotting, and allergic reactions
- Protects your nerves[34]

How to Benefit

Be sure to choose a reputable product, because there is a large difference between good- and poor-quality herbal products. It is best to choose either capsule or liquid form. If you're using capsules, choose products that are standardized to contain 24 percent ginkgo flavonoid glycosides. Take 120 mg of standardized extract per day, or a 40 mg capsule three times daily with meals. However, if you are suffering from a serious brain disease, supplement with 240 mg of ginkgo biloba extract daily for at least 3 months under professional guidance. Because the herb works to heal the brain and memory, it may take some time to see improvements; it is best taken consistently for several months, minimum. For ginkgo's preventive effects, 40 mg three times a day is ideal. If you're using a liquid extract, the standard dose is 30 to 60 drops three times daily.

Safety consideration: It's best to avoid fresh ginkgo leaves, because they contain some unwanted substances that may cause allergic reactions. (You won't be missing anything, because ginkgo is not the best-tasting herb.) Avoid products that have more than 5 parts per million of ginkgolic acid, which can cause allergic reactions. Avoid alcohol extracts if you are a recovering alcoholic or if you have liver disease.

Super Health Bonus

Ginkgo improves circulation throughout your body, so if you're suffering from cold hands or feet, you may notice an improvement while taking this herb. Some studies have attributed an aphrodisiac effect to ginkgo, probably due improved circulation throughout the body.[35] I can't speak to that effect, but in theory, it may work in this regard. Because of ginkgo's ability to deliver oxygen to your brain, it has also shown promise in the treatment of migraines.[36] In a preliminary study, ginkgo combined with vitamin C (ascorbic acid) was even able to assist in the reversal of memory and learning deficits caused by chronic fluoride exposure.[37] It is also believed that taking other herbal or nutritional supplements along with ginkgo helps deliver the substances to the brain, thanks to ginkgo's ability to improve brain circulation.[38]

60-SECOND BRAIN HEALTH TIP #50:
Make Magnesium Your Go-To Mineral

Low magnesium levels, a common occurrence, are linked to decreased cognitive function.

While many minerals are important to healthy brain functioning, magnesium is one of the most important ones. Based on his research at the

Mineral Element, Nutrition, Neuropsychological Function, and Behavior Research Lab at the Grand Forks Human Nutrition Research Center in North Dakota, James Penland, PhD, identifies magnesium as a critical mineral to maintain normal brain activity.[39]

A study published in *Procedures of the North Dakota Academy of Sciences* linked low magnesium intake to poorer scores on memory tests in rats. Other research links low magnesium levels to decreased cognitive function in humans.[40] Magnesium is involved with countless biological and chemical functions in the body, particularly in stabilizing brain-wave patterns and increasing blood flow to the brain.[41]

In their book, *The Magnesium Fac.....* Mildred S. Seelig, MD, MPH, and Andrea Rosanoff, PhD, fou..........sium deficiency is linked to many neurological concerns, incl.....

- Convulsions
- Hearing loss
- Hyperactivity, restlessness, ...vement
- Insomnia
- Migraines
- Numbness
- Tingling sensations in the bod....
- Tinnitus or a ringing sensation....
- Additionally, magnesium has been shown to prevent, treat, and reverse heart disease and high blood pressure, thereby playing a role in preventing strokes.[43]

While magnesium is critical to healthy brain function, few people get sufficient amounts of this mineral on an ongoing basis. Some experts estimate that as much as 80 percent of the population is deficient. Fortunately, addressing a deficiency can be as easy as eating more magnesium-rich foods and supplementing with the nutrient.

How to Benefit

Eat more magnesium-rich foods, which include nuts, legumes, whole grains, avocados, and artichokes. Additionally, supplement with 800 mg of magnesium glycinate or citrate daily. One of the best ways to obtain more magnesium is to apply it topically to your skin. Topical products usually contain magnesium chloride. Follow package directions for dosage amounts.

Super Health Bonus

Magnesium is essential for almost every function in your body. It is nature's stress reducer and relaxant. It boosts heart function, reduces arrhythmias, and relaxes muscles. Magnesium is helpful for leg cramps, as well.

60-SECOND BRAIN HEALTH TIP #51:

Pick Periwinkle: The Blue Flower for Gray Matter

Boost your short-term memory or treat dementia with this potent blue flower.

Not just for English gardens anymore, the lovely blue flowering plant periwinkle may help boost memory. Research shows that vinpocetine, a natural compound in periwinkle, helps transport oxygen and glucose to the brain. Since your brain needs both to function optimally, periwinkle may help prevent or treat brain disease.

With around 100 studies conducted on vinpocetine's effects on humans, mostly in Hungary, it is not surprising that it has been used by Hungarian doctors for 25 years to treat senility and blood vessel disorders in the brain. In these studies, it boosts memory and cognition in healthy people and in those with mild to moderate forms of dementia.

In a double-blind study published in the *European Journal of Clinical Pharmacology*, researchers tested vinpocetine's effect on the short-term memories of 12 healthy women. The women who took 40 mg of vinpocetine three times per day for 2 days scored 30 percent higher on short-term memory tests than the women in the placebo group.

In another double-blind study published in the journal *International Clinical Psychopharmacology,* researchers tested 165 people with mild to moderate dementia. After 16 weeks, 21 percent of those taking 30 to 60 mg of vinpocetine daily reported a decline in symptom severity, compared to only 7 percent of those taking the placebo.[44]

Vinpocetine is a potent free radical scavenger. Used regularly, it may help to prevent or slow senility and dementia by preventing free radicals from damaging the blood vessels in your brain. Vinpocetine also thins blood, boosts circulation to your brain, and improves your brain's ability to absorb nutrients, all of which improve brain function.[45] Research even shows that vinpocetine works as well as ginkgo biloba—an herbal superstar—for aiding brain oxygenation and improving cognitive abilities and memory.[46] To learn more about the brain benefits of ginkgo biloba, see 60-Second Brain Health Tip #49 on page 175.

Periwinkle and vinpocetine supplements show tremendous promise as a therapy for many brain diseases, especially stroke recovery. It is used in Europe and Japan as a natural therapy for stroke because it helps increase blood flow to areas of the brain with minimal function.[47]

How to Benefit

I typically suggest a dosage of 2 mg of periwinkle daily, taken with food. Vinpocetine appears to be safe for short- or long-term use. However, due to the compound's natural blood-thinning properties, it is a good idea to check with your doctor if you are taking blood-thinning medications; you may be able to reduce your dose of these medications while taking this supplement. If you have a serious brain disease, you may need a higher dosage. Experts suggest that doses of up to 10 mg daily may be helpful, but at that high dose you should be supervised by a qualified health-care professional. Unlike many nutritional supplements and herbs that need to build up in your body and take time to begin working, vinpocetine's effects tend to be fast acting.

Super Health Bonus

Vinpocetine has been found to increase energy in brain cells by improving your body's production of adenosine triphosphate (ATP), which is your body's primary cellular energy molecule. The increase in ATP production means you may experience improvement in conditions related to cellular energy production, such as chronic fatigue (long-standing fatigue) and chronic fatigue syndrome (a serious health condition involving many other symptoms in addition to fatigue).

60-SECOND BRAIN HEALTH TIP #52:
Recycle Brain-Healing Nutrients with Alpha Lipoic Acid

This powerful nutrient protects both the watery and the fatty parts of your brain from free radical damage.

A potent antioxidant called alpha lipoic acid, or sometimes just lipoic acid, offers tremendous help in treating existing brain diseases and in preventing the buildup of free radicals in your brain—a major contributing factor in most brain diseases. Being such a powerful antioxidant, it can help with maintaining overall brain health, as well.

Alpha lipoic acid is made by your body and found in every cell, including brain cells, where it assists with turning glucose into energy. Like all other antioxidants, it attacks brain-damaging free radicals. Unlike other antioxidants that work either in watery (vitamin C is an example) or fatty tissues (vitamin E is an example), alpha lipoic acid works equally well in both. That means it can work in the 60 percent of your brain that is fatty and the 40 percent of your brain that is watery. In other words, it is not limited in where it can protect your brain against harmful free radicals.

I may be alpha lipoic acid's biggest fan. After suffering a brain injury, a partially severed spinal cord, and resulting nerve damage in a car accident, I came upon alpha lipoic acid's brain and nerve health benefits almost accidentally. I had read about its antioxidant abilities nearly 20 years before and had started taking it just for its general health benefits, not really expecting to experience any difference. But I soon began noticing improvements in my pain and injuries, including improvement in the partial paralysis of my arm and a reduction in the eye pain linked to nerve damage. I can't say for sure whether alpha lipoic acid was the only factor at play, but I can say that it has become an essential part of my brain health repertoire—and that of many of my clients—over the years.

Perhaps part of alpha lipoic acid's tremendous power is its ability to readily cross the blood–brain barrier, where it can perform seemingly miraculous feats of healing. Few substances can actually cross this barrier to help with brain health, which is part of what makes alpha lipoic acid so amazing. Well, that and its potent free radical–scavenging capacity.[48] It literally seeks out and destroys free radicals before they can wreak havoc on your brain. This impressive nutrient also blocks some toxins' ability to damage your brain.

As if that weren't enough, alpha lipoic acid gives a helping hand to other brain antioxidants, including vitamins C and E and glutathione.[49] It literally works to recycle other antioxidant nutrients floating around your brain to keep them functioning long past their normal expiration date, allowing them to keep destroying brain-damaging free radicals. One of the world's preeminent alpha lipoic acid researchers, Lester Packer, PhD, director of the Packer Lab at the University of California at Berkeley, found that it may offer powerful protection against stroke (and heart disease in general). He describes it as "the most versatile and powerful antioxidant in the entire antioxidant defense network."[50]

Alpha lipoic acid also appears to help boost memory. A study conducted at the Clinical Institute for Mental Health in Mannheim, Germany, explored the effects of alpha lipoic acid on memory loss in aging mice, since they experience aging-related memory issues similar to those of humans. The mice were divided into groups: those that were given alpha lipoic acid in their water and those that drank water with nothing else in it. After 2 weeks, the mice were placed in a maze to determine how well they could navigate their way through it. Mice treated with alpha lipoic acid performed much better than untreated mice half their age. The researchers speculated that the alpha lipoic acid reduced the free radical damage in the brains of those mice and perhaps even slowed the age-related loss of brain cells. More studies on alpha lipoic acid's specific memory-improving abilities will undoubtedly help to determine the exact mechanisms by which it improves memory. In the meantime, there has definitely been enough research to start benefiting from the nutrient's brain-protective powers.

High doses of alpha lipoic acid have also been found to slow the progression of multiple sclerosis in animal experiments.[51] And when it comes to stroke and brain injuries, alpha lipoic acid is seemingly unmatched in its abilities. Dr. Packer found in his studies that alpha lipoic acid produced spectacular results in animals that had suffered from a stroke, and even showed that it can completely prevent stroke-related brain damage. He says, "If lipoic acid can prevent brain injury during an acute free radical attack, such as that experienced during a stroke, then I believe over time it will protect the brain from the free radical attack normally experienced every day."[52]

How to Benefit

Alpha lipoic acid is available in capsule or tablet form. It is known by a variety of names, including alpha lipoic acid; thioctic acid; and 1, 2 dithiolane-3-pentanoic acid, although alpha lipoic acid is increasingly becoming the standard name. While it is sometimes shortened to ALA (which is actually incorrect), keep in mind that it is not the same as alpha linolenic acid, which is a type of fat. Occasionally, alpha lipoic acid may be sold under the name alpha lipotene.

I usually recommend a dose of 100 mg daily. It is a cousin of the B vitamin biotin and can compete with biotin if taken in high doses, so if you're taking more than 100 mg daily (as is often beneficial in brain disease), you should supplement with biotin, as well. Ideally, take 50 mg of alpha lipoic acid in the morning and 50 mg in the evening so its antioxidant activities continue throughout the day and night.

Super Health Bonus

You may notice that your immune system is stronger while supplementing with alpha lipoic acid. That's because it has powerful immune-boosting properties. It has even prevented the replication of the HIV virus in human cells in a test tube.

60-SECOND BRAIN HEALTH TIP #53:
Seek a Wise Sage

Boost your mood and short- and long-term memory with sage oil.

When it comes to brain health and mental acuity, few people think of herbs. While Mother Nature's herbal medicines humbly lie upon the earth in her rain forests, wilderness areas, and jungles devoid of any slick advertising campaigns, they show tremendous promise in the prevention of brain diseases and in maintaining great brain health. And sage is one of the best examples.

Sage is a great all-natural brain health remedy. As early as 1597, herbalists wrote that sage "is singularly good for the head and brain and quickeneth the nerves and memory." In 1652, well-known herbalist Nicholas Culpepper wrote that sage "heals the memory, warming and quickening the senses," and it appears these herbalists were right.

A British research team conducted a study of sage's therapeutic properties on a group of 44 adults between the ages of 18 and 37. Some participants were given capsules of sage oil while others were given a placebo of sunflower oil. Results showed that those who took the sage oil performed significantly better at memory tests than those who took the placebo. The people who were given sage as part of the study had improvements in both immediate and delayed word recall scores, as well as mood improvements. Additional research by the same scientific team led them to conclude that sage may also be helpful for those suffering from Alzheimer's disease.[53]

While sage is showing promise in the treatment of brain diseases, it also has benefits for healthy individuals who wish to maintain a healthy brain. In other research, a number of significant effects on cognition were noted with the sage species *Salvia lavandulifolia*. The effects included improvements in both immediate and delayed word recall scores. The researchers concluded that sage oil is capable of affecting mood and cognition in healthy young adults.[54] This team found that sage inhibits the enzyme acetylcholinesterase (AChE). AChE breaks down the neurotransmitter acetylcholine, which plays an important role in healthy communication between brain cells. Acetylcholine is essential to mood regulation and brain–muscle coordination, as well as the formation of new memories. It tends to be depleted in patients with Alzheimer's disease.[55]

Additional research suggests that one or more constituents of *S. lavandulifolia*, when taken orally, cross the gastrointestinal and blood–brain barriers to reach the brain and may inhibit a potentially brain-damaging substance called cholinesterase in select areas of the brain.[56]

The German Ministry of Health is currently considering updating its Commission E Monographs—a compilation of the safety and effectiveness of herbs—to add sage as a treatment for Alzheimer's disease. While there are various species of sage, the one most commonly used in memory studies is *S. lavandulifolia*.

How to Benefit

Fresh sage is an excellent addition to soups, stews, and chicken dishes. Add it toward the end of the cooking time, because excessive cooking can damage some of the therapeutic compounds found in fresh sage. While sage is most commonly available as a dried herb, most of the study benefits were achieved by taking sage oil capsules from the *S. lavandulifolia* plant. Because oil constituents vary by brand, follow package directions. Most health food stores also sell dried sage that can be used for cooking or for tea. To make sage tea, use 1 teaspoon of dried herb per cup of hot water. Allow it to steep for 10 to 15 minutes before drinking, and enjoy a cup two or three times daily.

Remember that herbs are potent medicines, so to prevent drug–herb interactions, it is important to consult with your doctor before you start taking any.

Super Health Bonus

Germany already recognizes sage as a treatment for dyspepsia, excessive perspiration, and inflammation of the mouth and nose, so if you're experiencing any of these health conditions, you'll probably see an improvement alongside improved memory.

60-SECOND BRAIN HEALTH TIP #54:
Sniff Lavender for a Mood Boost

Conquer depression with the flower that has proven itself more effective than antidepressant drugs.

Not just a beautiful scent, lavender is also proven to reduce anxiety and depression and may help balance brain hormones for improved mood.

I visited an organic lavender farm last summer. About half a mile down the road, I knew I was close, as I could smell the fragrance wafting through the air. The rolling hillside was full of stunning, silvery green and purple lavender plants. While I've never been to France, I imagine this is what the French countryside must look and smell like. I felt immediately transported to a peaceful place. How much was linked to the actual aromatic effects of lavender or the natural beauty of it in this lovely environment, I'll never know. Either way, it was an experience to remember.

Lavender has been in use for at least 2,500 years, since a time when it was applied to mummification and perfume making by the ancient Egyptians, Phoenicians, and Arabs. Ancient Romans are also believed to have used lavender for cooking, bathing, and scenting the air. New research shows that these ancient civilizations were on to something when they incorporated lavender flowers into their day-to-day lives. We now know that lavender can alleviate anxiety and depression, most likely by balancing neurotransmitters in the brain.

In a study comparing the effects of a medication for depression to the effects of drinking tea made from lavender flowers, participants drank 2 cups each day of an infusion made with lavender. The scientists found that the lavender was slightly more effective than the antidepressant drugs. The researchers concluded that lavender might be used as an adjunct to antidepressant drugs or on its own to assist with symptoms of depression.[57]

As you learned in 60-Second Brain Health Tip #32 on page 129, getting a good night's sleep is imperative to brain health. Lavender can also help ensure that your sleep is restorative and brain healing. Lavender is an excellent insomnia remedy. According to James Duke, PhD, botanist and author of *The Green Pharmacy*, British hospitals used lavender essential oil in patients' baths or sprinkled onto their bedclothes to help them sleep.[58]

How to Benefit

To obtain the study-proven antidepressant effects, drink 2 cups of lavender flower tea daily. To make lavender tea, add 2 teaspoons of dried flowers to boiled water and let it steep for 10 minutes. Strain and drink. Of course, never discontinue any antidepressant medications without consulting your physician.

To use in a bath to help you get a good night's sleep, sprinkle 5 to 10 drops of lavender essential oil under the running water as the tub fills, to allow the oils to disperse. Alternatively, place a heaping tablespoon of dried lavender flowers in cheesecloth, tie into a bundle, and allow it to infuse the bathwater while soaking.

You can also find lavender water in some health food stores or online. You can spray the lavender water directly on your pillow or sheets to help you get brain-restorative sleep each night. Be aware that if you use lavender essential oil, it may stain your bedding, so lavender water, also known as lavender hydrosol, is preferable.

Super Health Bonus

For women who may be suffering from premenstrual syndrome (PMS), research shows that lavender is helpful for reducing emotional issues attributed to monthly hormonal fluctuations. A study published in the journal *BioPsycho-Social Medicine* found that inhaling the scent of lavender for 10 minutes had a significant effect on the nervous systems of women suffering from premenstrual symptoms. It especially decreased feelings of depression and confusion linked to PMS. To alleviate mood-related PMS symptoms, place a few drops of lavender essential oil on a handkerchief and inhale periodically. You can also make a tea from dried lavender flowers, as described above, or simply breathe in the aroma of a lavender plant growing indoors or outdoors.[59]

60-SECOND BRAIN HEALTH TIP #55:
Pick Curcumin for a Better Brain

Give your brain a significant memory boost within an hour of taking this potent nutrient.

By now you may already be enjoying the brain health benefits of curries, complete with the spice turmeric. But supplementing with curcumin, one of the active ingredients in turmeric, is another powerful way to protect your brain from disease. Research conducted by Greg Cole, PhD, associate director of the Mary S. Easton Center for Alzheimer's Disease Research at UCLA, showed that curcumin, the yellow pigment in turmeric, is a potent weapon against inflammation and plaque buildup in the brain.[60] As we've discussed, inflammation and plaque have been linked to serious brain diseases, including Alzheimer's. Additional studies are having similar positive results.

University of British Columbia researcher Patrick McGeer and Sun Health Research Institute, Arizona, researcher Jo Rogers found that arthritis patients treated with anti-inflammatory drugs were seven times less likely to develop Alzheimer's disease. From that connection, they found some of the earliest evidence of a link between Alzheimer's disease and inflammation. Prior to that research, we didn't know that Alzheimer's disease was linked to chronic inflammation.

Strong arthritis drugs aren't a great option for most Alzheimer's patients, as they are linked with serious side effects. While some of these drugs, known as COX-2 inhibitors, have been pulled from the market due to the deaths linked to them, many are back again. To my knowledge, there weren't any formulation changes with these drugs, so additional deaths are likely.

Fortunately, curcumin is an all-natural COX-2 inhibitor. Unlike the deadly drugs, it works on an additional level of inflammation and lacks the negative side effects. Prostaglandins are chemical messengers that are frequently responsible for inflammation in the body. They are made by two enzymes known as cyclooxygenase-1 (COX-1) and cyclooxygenase-2 (COX-2). While the arthritis drugs seem to work on the COX-2 enzymes alone, turmeric works on both enzymes to stop inflammation in its tracks. Even better: Curcumin has shown promise in the treatment of many serious diseases. You may actually experience many *positive* side effects of supplementing with it on a regular basis.

As you may recall from Chapter 4, where we discussed the brain benefits of choosing turmeric, research conducted by a medical team at a graduate school at Kanazawa University, Japan, demonstrated that curcumin, found in turmeric, prevents the development of a substance called beta amyloid in the brain. This substance is a causative factor for Alzheimer's disease.[61] Additionally, an animal study published in the *Journal of Neuroscience Research* found that the brain-boosting curcumin could improve spatial learning and memory.[62]

As we also discussed in Chapter 4, even Alzheimer's patients with severe symptoms, including dementia, irritability, agitation, anxiety, and apathy, showed excellent therapeutic results when taking curcumin. When they took 764 mg of turmeric with a standardized amount of 100 mg of curcumin every day for 12 weeks, they "started recovering from these symptoms without any adverse reaction in the clinical symptom and laboratory data." After

3 months of treatment, the patients' symptoms and their reliance on caregivers significantly decreased. After 1 year of treatment, two of the patients recognized their family members, although they were unable to do so at the outset of the study. In one of the cases, the person had a 17 percent improvement on their mini-mental state examination (MMSE) score.[63] While the study size was small, the promising results were still impressive. Additional research into curcumin as a treatment option for Alzheimer's disease holds great promise.

How to Benefit

Both turmeric and curcumin supplements are readily available in most health food stores or from your natural health professional. If you choose to take turmeric, I recommend taking 1 to 3 grams of the dried, powdered root daily. The supplement package should indicate how much of the dried root is found in each capsule or tablet. Most people find capsules easier to digest. For brain disease prevention and treatment, I prefer a standardized curcumin supplement. Take 400 mg of curcumin three times daily, for a total of 1,200 mg per day.

Super Health Bonus

In addition to the many brain health benefits of supplementing with curcumin, the nutrient is also a powerful fat-reducing formula that appears to work in seven different ways. Research in *PLoS One* shows that curcumin effectively decreases inflammatory compounds in fat stores linked to fat hoarding.[64] So don't be surprised if you lose some excess weight and experience fewer cravings, because curcumin also has a proven ability to balance blood sugar levels, and stable levels tend to reduce cravings, mood swings, and energy dips. Curcumin has also been shown to fight infections and even have anticancer properties, making it potentially beneficial in the prevention or treatment of some cancers.

60-SECOND BRAIN HEALTH TIP #56:
Seize Fish Oil Supplements for Superior Intellect

Give yourself a bigger, more resilient brain with fish oil supplements.

The verdict is in: Fish eaters have bigger, better, more resilient brains. On average, the difference between fish eaters and those who don't eat fish is significant. Fish eaters have a 14 percent larger hippocampus, which is the biggest part of your brain, involved with memory and learning. They also have a 4 percent larger frontal orbital cortex, which is the part of your brain involved in executive function. And that's not all: Fish eaters also have a reduced risk of Alzheimer's disease and a slowing of cognitive decline.[65]

But what if you want the brain benefits of eating fish without actually eating fish? Let's face it: Fish isn't to everyone's liking. Thanks to the creation of fish oil and docosahexaenoic acid (DHA) supplements derived from cold-water fish, you can get the benefits of eating fish without ever hitting the local sushi bar.

Of course, I still encourage you to eat fish on a regular basis—at least weekly, but preferably a few times a week—to obtain the big brain benefits of doing so. In a study of people who ate fish three times a month, researchers found that they had a 40 percent reduced risk of suffering from Alzheimer's disease in comparison to people who never ate fish.[66] The *Journal of Molecular Neuroscience* also showed that increasing your intake of DHA, which is one of the key nutrients found in fish oils, could actually reverse some of the mental decline associated with Alzheimer's disease.[67] Most brain experts consider mental decline linked with Alzheimer's to be irreversible, so these findings are significant.

And if that wasn't enough, researchers found that mice fed a diet rich in DHA had a whopping 70 percent less amyloid protein—the type that forms plaques implicated in Alzheimer's disease—after only 5 months.[68] That's astounding. I'm not aware of any drug that can even compare to this result.

How to Benefit

Look for a fish oil, DHA, or combination DHA and eicosapentaenoic acid (EPA) supplement that is confirmed by third-party laboratory results to be free of mercury. I prefer a combination DHA and EPA supplement because your brain needs both of these fats for maximum health. There's great news for people who are deficient in these nutrients, too: People who are deficient in omega-3 fatty acids (DHA and EPA are two types of omega-3s) absorb twice as many fatty acids once they start supplementing with them, compared with people who already have sufficient amounts. That's your body's wisdom at work to correct an imbalance and restore brain and overall bodily health.

Take two capsules of 1,000 mg of fish oils daily. Each capsule should contain at least 180 mg of EPA and 120 mg of DHA, for best results. They are best taken with food to increase absorption and to reduce the fishy aftertaste that some people experience. If you take them with food and still have gas and a fishy aftertaste, you may be deficient in the enzyme lipase, which is needed to digest fats. If so, simply take a full-spectrum digestive enzyme formula that contains lipase with your fish oil or DHA-EPA supplements.

Super Health Bonus

Omega-3 fatty acids such as DHA and EPA, found in fish oil supplements, also protect your heart against heart disease, so you'll reduce your risk of brain and heart diseases simultaneously. Plus, they've been shown to help restore a healthy body weight and boost immunity.

60-SECOND BRAIN HEALTH TIP #57:
Gain New Hope for Parkinson's Disease with Gastrodin

This natural supplement, derived from Chinese orchids, treats headaches, stroke, and even Parkinson's disease.

Environmental pollutants and frequent stressors can expedite normal aging processes.[69,70] Fortunately, your brain cells have systems in place to defend themselves against these ongoing threats.[71] Exciting new research shows that your brain has the capacity to preserve and protect brain cells.[72] Perhaps even more exciting, researchers have isolated a compound known as gastrodin from Chinese orchids (*Gastrodia elata*). These orchids have been used in traditional Chinese medicine to treat dizziness, headaches, and stroke and are now known to strongly bolster your brain's natural defenses and regenerative mechanisms.[73]

Gastrodin has been found to be a potent brain cell protector in studies in four journals: the *Journal of Traditional Chinese Medicine*, the *International Journal of Biochemistry and Molecular Biology*, the *Journal of Pharmacy and Pharmacology*, and *Neurochemistry International*.

While it is still in the experimental stages for the possible treatment of Parkinson's disease in animals, exciting research in the journal *Life Sciences* found that gastrodin blocked diseased brain pathways involved in Parkinson's and may offer new hope for treatment.[74]

Gastrodin has also been found to be helpful in the treatment of stroke. In a study by the Institute of Geriatrics at Beijing University of Chinese Medicine, researchers found that gastrodin was similar to Duxil (a drug used to treat stroke) in its effects on mild to moderate dementia caused by heart disease or small strokes in the brain.[75]

According to research, gastrodin works on multiple levels.

1. It supports normal, healthy levels of blood flow in humans and animals.[76]

2. It helps maintain healthy levels of essential neurotransmitters—the brain's chemical messengers.[77]

3. It helps support the body's defenses against aging-related mild memory problems.[78]

4. It reduces the effects of everyday stresses and tensions.[79]

How to Benefit

While Chinese orchid has been used for many years in traditional Chinese medicine, the standardized extract of gastrodin is a fairly new and cutting-edge supplement. Life Extension is one of the primary, if not the only, manufacturer of gastrodin, which is produced under the product name Brain Shield. Take 300 mg of gastrodin twice daily for brain support. Parkinson's patients may need higher doses than that but should work with a qualified herbalist in conjunction with their neurologist before taking this supplement. After 1 month, reduce your dosage to 300 mg once daily.

Super Health Bonus

Taking gastrodin on a daily basis may do more than prevent brain diseases and potentially treat stroke and Parkinson's disease; it may also reduce the frequency of headaches, which is the customary use for Chinese orchid in traditional Chinese medicine.

60-SECOND BRAIN HEALTH TIP #58:
Select Cordyceps to Prevent and Treat Stroke

Prevent and treat stroke with the medicinal mushroom proven to boost learning and memory, too.

The mushroom cordyceps has been widely used in traditional Chinese medicine to combat the effects of aging. And now research is proving the effectiveness of this natural supplement. Cordyceps contains an active ingredient identified as cordycepin, which has been shown to improve learning and memory.

According to a study published in the *European Journal of Pharmacology*, researchers found that cordycepin helps improve cognition in animals and may be beneficial in the treatment of stroke.[80] Based on research in the *Journal of Medicinal Food*, cordyceps acts as a potent antioxidant and even has the ability to improve memory impairment.[81] The antioxidant and healing effects of cordyceps were significantly beneficial in both the prevention and treatment of stroke.[82]

Cordyceps works to prevent and treat stroke primarily by reducing brain-damaging free radicals. One of the ways the mushroom is able to do this is by boosting your body's own production of superoxide dismutase.[83] This specialized protein, known as an enzyme, is also one of the most potent antioxidants in your body and helps to protect against brain diseases.

Additional research in the *European Journal of Pharmacology* found that cordycepin lowered the inflammatory compound known as MMP-3 (matrix metalloproteinase-3), which tends to be elevated after the occurrence of stroke.[84] The same study also found that cordyceps demonstrates anticancer activity and may be helpful in the prevention or treatment of brain cancer. Further research will help to determine the effectiveness of cordyceps against brain cancer.

Cordyceps was also shown to have general memory-enhancing effects in a study published in the journal *Archives of Pharmacal Research*.[85]

How to Benefit

Cordyceps supplements come in both powder and capsule forms. Choose a 5:1 extract from organically grown and processed cordyceps mushrooms to ensure sufficient potency to reap the brain-boosting effects. Take 600 mg daily for general brain health, as well as stroke prevention and healing. This dose also has demonstrated potential effectiveness against brain cancer.

Choose a brand that has undergone laboratory testing to show it is free of heavy metals and microbial contaminants. I particularly like Herb's Best Nutrition brand, which has this certification, is made from organic mushrooms, and has a high potency. Visit my Web site, DrMichelleCook.com, to learn more about cordyceps and this product.

Super Health Bonus

Cordyceps is also an immune-boosting and energizing medicinal mushroom that has many other therapeutic effects, including helping to prevent cancer and reducing the damaging effects of stress on the body. Many herbalists, myself included, use cordyceps on a regular basis to give the immune system a boost when people are under significant stress or are dealing with cancer. Don't be surprised if you have fewer colds or flus along with greater energy while taking this supplement.

60-SECOND BRAIN HEALTH TIP #59:
Race for Brilliance with Reishi Mushrooms

Protect your brain from seizures, Huntington's disease, and stroke damage with this amazing medicinal mushroom.

In the previous 60-Second Brain Health Tip, you discovered the brain-boosting power of cordyceps. But cordyceps isn't the only medicinal mushroom that is showing huge promise in building memory and preventing and treating brain diseases. Reishi mushrooms, which have also long been used in traditional Chinese medicine, are getting great brain health results, too. According to research in the *International Journal of Medicinal Mushrooms*, reishi mushrooms protect brain and nerve cells and even reduce seizures in animals prone to them.[86]

Even more impressive, reishi is showing huge promise as a possible treatment for Huntington's disease.[87] Huntington's disease is a serious degenerative brain disorder that affects muscles, memory, and behavior patterns of people suffering from the illness. While the research into reishi's effectiveness against the disease is still in its infancy, anything that shows promise as a treatment for such a serious illness is welcome, particularly natural options that lack the horrific side effects linked to many pharmaceutical drugs. Reishi appears to work on the pathways that regulate the energy centers of brain cells.[88]

Like the medicinal mushroom cordyceps, reishi has also been found in studies to protect the brain against free radical damage, including damage from stroke.[89]

How to Benefit

Medicinal mushrooms like reishi come in both powder and capsule forms. Take 300 mg of organically grown and organically processed reishi daily for general brain health, stroke prevention and healing, and possible protection against Huntington's disease.

As with other medicinal mushroom supplements, be sure the brand you choose is independently certified to be free of heavy metals and microbial contaminants. Visit my Web site at DrMichelleCook.com for more information.

Super Health Bonus

Like cordyceps, reishi is an immune-boosting and energizing medicinal mushroom that has many other therapeutic effects, including reducing the damaging effects of stress on your body. Many herbalists, myself included, use reishi on a regular basis to give the immune system a boost when people are under significant stress, particularly if they feel exhausted mentally and physically. Don't be surprised if you have fewer colds or flus along with greater energy while taking either or both of these supplements.

Brain Power in Action Success Tips

As you head into the eating part of the plan, the following tips from the test panelists will keep you inspired and on track.

"My first week was good. I didn't follow the eating program 100 percent (probably more like 60 percent, if not a bit more). But I am adding more healthy things daily, and I am taking the supplements. I feel better already. Without even realizing it, my energy was up after work, so I got some things done that I normally would try to do over the weekend."

—Dawn Field

"So far this week I've added multivitamins, B-complex vitamins, ginkgo biloba, and omega-3 supplements to my pharmacopeia. I've cut way down on sugar (no chocolate!) and reduced my meat and dairy intake. I still have a little low-fat milk in my oatmeal (with flaxseed!) and coffee. As a happy result, I no longer call the dogs by my kids' names."

—Mitch Mandel

"I slipped last night at my sister's Halloween party. I didn't eat candy, but I did eat a sandwich and some tortilla chips with guacamole along with a small cup of punch. Back on track today! Surprisingly, my daughter's candy doesn't even sound good to me."

—Renee Carter

"I couldn't find anything to add to my salad at lunchtime today, so for the first time, I cooked some tofu in olive oil and mixed it in with my salad. It was surprisingly delicious!"

—Janine Lewis

"At some point all of us will have one of those days and slip up. Don't be hard on yourself. I think the point of this is to make mini lifestyle changes. Celebrate any positive changes you've made over the course of the week and forgive yourself for the slipups. I didn't have a perfect first week, but I did make several positive changes!"

—Donna Cervac

PART III

BRAIN-BOOSTING RECIPES

The Basics

Breakfasts and Bread

Beverages

Appetizers, Dips, and Spreads

Soups and Stews

Salads and Salad Dressings

Entrées

Desserts

THE BASICS

Some of the common reasons people tell me they don't eat better include "I don't have time," "It's too much work," or "It costs too much." The reality is that with some added knowledge, it takes very little time, effort, or money to eat well, and the result is greater energy and brain health to do all the other things you want to do. Once you get started on this way of eating to super-charge your brain, you'll quickly discover it increases your time by increasing your energy. And as for cost, after ditching most prepared, packaged, and processed foods, you'll likely find that your grocery bill drops. With a few basics under your belt, you'll be amazed at how simple, inexpensive, and rewarding this way of eating can be even if you're on the road, have young children, have an intense career, or just have a busy life. And isn't that just about everyone these days?

Stocking Your Kitchen

While you really don't need any special equipment to prepare a bountiful, brain-boosting banquet, a few handy items will make following this program easy for life. Of course, it's not necessary to give up on the whole program if you don't have these items or the money to purchase them. You can still do marvelously well with nothing more than a knife, cutting board, pan, and a bowl or two, which almost everyone has readily available.

Because eating more delicious greens and gourmet salads is such a valuable component of the *60 Seconds to Boost Your Brain Power* program, you may wish to get a good salad spinner, since they can make light work of cleaning and drying greens. You can purchase a good-quality one for about $20 or less. Alternatively, you can choose prewashed greens.

You can add a juicer, food processor, and blender as you are able, to minimize your effort and maximize your results. If you wish to add another small appliance, I suggest a good-quality ice cream maker. I've included a few ice cream recipes since almost everyone loves ice cream. If you don't have an ice cream maker, that's no problem. Just pour the blended ice cream recipe into ice pop molds for delicious, creamy pops.

Food Processor

A food processor makes light work of chopping, mincing, grating, slicing, and mixing. In seconds it can complete what might take many minutes to do manually, thereby making it a snap to complete the recipes when you're short on time. There are many good-quality ones on the market at affordable prices.

Juice It Up

The idea of juicing fresh fruits and vegetables first started with a man named Norman Walker. Born in 1875, he was recovering from health problems in the French countryside. While observing the women in the kitchen peeling carrots, he noticed how moist the vegetables were beneath the skin. He had the idea that grinding them up to release the juice would help him recover his health, which proved to be accurate. Later, he moved to California, where he and a medical doctor friend opened a juice bar, concocting fresh juices for specific health conditions. And the fresh juice craze had begun in North America. He probably played a significant role in shaping California into the health-conscious state it is today.

With minimal effort, you can juice at home. Of course, a juicer is not an essential part of the *60 Seconds to Boost Your Brain Power* program, but it is a great addition and is highly recommended. Freshly made vegetable and fruit juices pack a ton of nutrition in every sip.

There are many different kinds of juicers, ranging from $40 to more than $1,000. It's not necessary to buy a high-end juicer to reap the benefits. I always tell people the best juicer is the one you will use. If a steep price tag is an excuse not to purchase a juicer, get an inexpensive one. Most of the popular kitchen appliance manufacturers offer models that use a spinning technique;

these are called centrifugal juicers. While these types also spin air into the juice that may cause it to oxidize faster, they're still better than no juicer at all. The more expensive juicers are usually called masticating juicers and tend to spin the juice more slowly, thereby increasing the amount of fiber, vitamins, and minerals you'll get in your juice. Many of these juicers are multipurpose, enabling you to make fruit or vegetable purees, baby food, fresh nut butters, and healthy frozen desserts. You can also make "total juice" or "whole juice" in a high-powered blender, which I'll explain momentarily.

There are also juicers specifically suited for citrus fruits like lemons, limes, oranges, and grapefruits. Some are as basic as a wooden or ceramic reamer that you push into half of the fruit and turn while holding the fruit over a pitcher or bowl. Other options are fully electric, requiring you to press half of the citrus fruit down against a spinning reamer. These range from plastic versions typically costing $25 to $35 to stainless steel ones typically costing $150 to $175. I've used both electric and manual ones and actually prefer the inexpensive ceramic type that sits on the counter and has a handle to hold while you press the citrus fruit with the other hand. (For convenience, find one that has a small bowl to hold the juice.) I then pour the juice through a strainer to remove pulp and seeds that may have found their way into the juice.

Blenders

My husband's and my birthdays are only a day apart, so a decade and a half ago we decided to buy a Vitamix blender as a joint birthday gift. It lasted 12 years with heavy-duty daily use and was one of the best investments we've made for our health. We've since replaced it with a newer model. Rarely does a day go by that we don't use it. It gets a serious workout in the creation of healthy and delicious soups, smoothies, frappés, total juices, almond milk, and other healthy creations. A high-powered blender like the Vitamix has the capacity to do much more than other blenders, but its price tag tends to be a bit steep—in the $400 to $650 range, depending on the model. However, as

I stated for juicers, it's not essential to buy a top-of-the-line model. If you have a standard blender, you can still make most, if not all, of the recipes that follow. And most blenders cost less than $50.

The Traveling Brainiac

It's possible to have your frequent-flyer miles and your brain health, too. With a little planning, you'll continue to reap the benefits of reduced inflammation, a healthier brain, improved energy levels, and delicious healthy foods. Here are some simple tips.

1. When traveling via plane or train, call in advance to check if a fruit plate or salad is available on board. Many airlines and rail companies offer these healthier options.

2. Bring pieces of fruit or veggie sticks on car or bus trips should you have difficulty finding healthy options along the way.

3. Choose a salad in restaurants. Simply ask for some lemon wedges and olive oil instead of dressing. Most restaurants are happy to accommodate this request. Most high-quality restaurants offer mixed green salads with leafy greens that actually resemble their name, but if the restaurant calls iceberg lettuce a "green salad," just ask to have it topped off with cucumber slices, green or red bell peppers, and tomatoes to increase its nutritional value.

4. Many international restaurants offer better options than those that offer only standard North American fare. Middle Eastern (Lebanese, Turkish, Iranian, Iraqi, Egyptian), Greek, Mexican, and Asian (Japanese, Thai, and some Chinese) restaurants are often likely to serve more vegetables, beans, and whole grains than the typical burger and fry joints. Be sure to avoid Asian sauces if you're choosing Japanese, Thai, or Chinese food, as they frequently contain monosodium glutamate (MSG) even when the restaurateur insists otherwise.

5. Raw nuts and seeds are excellent choices while traveling, since they offer a high amount of protein and essential fatty acids and help keep blood sugar levels stable, thereby warding off cravings for unhealthy items.

6. Check the Internet or local phone books to find out if there are any organic markets, health food stores, or healthy restaurants in the areas where you'll be staying.

It takes some effort to eat healthier when you're on the road or in the skies, but the effort is definitely rewarded in the form of better brain health.

Here are some of my favorite brain-boosting recipes. You'll soon discover that you won't feel deprived on this program, as it is packed with delicious foods. I included breakfast options, since people often tell me they don't know what to choose for a healthy breakfast. And, of course, there are also many amazing dessert recipes.

BLUEBERRY PANCAKES

These delicious pancakes are high in fiber and calcium and make a great brain-boosting breakfast, thanks particularly to the blueberries they are topped with. They're so simple to whip up from scratch that you'll wonder why you ever bothered with mixes. Plus they taste substantially better.

MAKES 2 TO 4 SERVINGS

1 cup almond flour

½ cup tapioca flour or arrowroot flour

1½ teaspoons aluminum-free baking powder

1 tablespoon raw sugar

1 egg

1 cup soy milk

Coconut oil

1–2 cups fresh or frozen and thawed blueberries

In a medium bowl, mix the flours, baking powder, and sugar. Add the egg and soy milk and whisk until combined.

In a medium skillet over medium heat, melt the coconut oil. Pour or scoop the pancake batter into the skillet.

Cook for 2 to 3 minutes. After most of the bubbles break, flip the pancakes and cook the other sides for 2 minutes longer. Serve immediately.

Top with the blueberries.

BRAIN-BUILDING EGGLESS SCRAMBLE

I am frequently asked for ways to add more brain-healing turmeric to a diet. This recipe is an easy and delicious way to do that. Turmeric's natural anti-inflammatory properties help reduce low-grade inflammation in your brain and body. Plus this dish is loaded with nutrients and fiber from the vegetables and high in protein and calcium, making it a great substitute for traditional scrambled eggs. It also makes a quick and delicious dinner.

MAKES 4 SERVINGS

8 ounces firm tofu, crumbled

1 teaspoon ground turmeric

1 teaspoon unrefined sea salt

½ teaspoon ground cumin (optional, but a delicious addition)

4 tomatoes, cored and quartered

2 tablespoons extra-virgin olive oil

1 large onion, chopped

2 ribs celery, chopped

1 red bell pepper, chopped

In a medium bowl, combine the tofu, turmeric, salt, and cumin, if using.

In a blender or food processor, puree the tomatoes.

In a large skillet over medium-low heat, heat the oil, making sure it doesn't smoke. Add the onion and cook, stirring frequently, for 5 to 10 minutes or until softened. Add the celery and red pepper and cook, stirring frequently, for 5 minutes or until tender. Add the seasoned tofu and cook until heated through. Stir in the tomato puree, cover, and cook for 5 to 10 minutes or until heated through and the flavors have blended.

SUPERBRAINIAC BREAKFAST SMOOTHIE

My mom developed this breakfast smoothie to have in place of coffee when she wants to jump-start her day. It's packed with vitamins, minerals, and fiber. The berries or purple grapes not only add delicious flavor, they offer important brain-boosting proanthocyanidins and resveratrol, respectively.

MAKES 1 OR 2 SERVINGS

1 banana

1 tablespoon ground flaxseeds or ground chia seeds

1 tablespoon green powder (such as spirulina or chlorella) or 1 cup fresh spinach or other leafy green

1 teaspoon coconut oil

1½ cups frozen fruit (blueberries, strawberries, or purple grapes)

2 cups water

In a blender, combine the banana, seeds, green powder or spinach or leafy green, oil, fruit, and 1½ cups of the water. Blend until smooth. Add the remaining ½ cup of water, if desired, until the smoothie reaches desired consistency. Drink immediately.

SOY FRUIT SMOOTHIE

This refreshing smoothie affords an easy way to enjoy a quick breakfast.
When strawberries are not in season, frozen berries will work just as well.

MAKES 2 SERVINGS

2 cups calcium-fortified vanilla
  soy milk, well chilled

1 cup sliced frozen peaches

1 banana, cut into chunks

8 strawberries

¼ teaspoon ground cinnamon

Ice cubes (optional)

In a blender, combine the soy milk, peaches, banana, strawberries, and cinnamon. Pulse until smooth and creamy. Add a few ice cubes, if desired, and blend again.

GREEN TEA AND BLUEBERRY SMOOTHIE

While this smoothie provides an extra boost of antioxidants from the green tea, you don't need to worry about becoming jittery on this small amount of caffeine in the morning. If time is a concern, brew your tea and mix in the honey the night before. Refrigerate until morning, and your smoothie will be ready in just a few minutes.

MAKES 2 SERVINGS

3 tablespoons boiling water

1 green tea bag

2 teaspoons honey

1½ cups frozen blueberries

½ banana

¾ cup calcium-fortified light vanilla soy milk

In a heatproof cup, pour the boiling water over the tea bag and allow to steep for 3 minutes. Remove the tea bag. Stir the honey into the tea until it dissolves. In a blender with ice-crushing ability, combine the blueberries, banana, soy milk, and tea. Blend on the highest setting until smooth. (Some blenders may require additional water to process the mixture.) Divide between 2 tall glasses and serve.

ORANGE AND DRIED CHERRY PORRIDGE

Millet is a small, round grain that is easily digested and easy on your blood sugar. It is loaded with fiber and B-complex vitamins. Toasting the millet for a few minutes brings out its nutty, mild flavor.

MAKES 4 SERVINGS

⅔ cup millet

2 cups water

½ cup orange juice

½ cup dried cherries

2 tablespoons coconut sugar

¼ teaspoon ground allspice

1 cup calcium-fortified soy milk

½ cup chopped pistachios

In a dry saucepan over medium heat, toast the millet for 3 minutes, stirring often, or until the millet is fragrant and just begins to pop. Gradually stir in the water, orange juice, cherries, sugar, and allspice and bring to a boil. Reduce the heat to low, cover, and cook, stirring occasionally, for 25 to 30 minutes, or until the millet is tender and the liquid is absorbed. Stir in the soy milk and heat through. Top each serving with 2 tablespoons of the pistachios.

APPLE-CINNAMON-WALNUT OATS

This is a quick and hot breakfast for those chilly winter mornings. The cinnamon and the fiber in the oats and apple help ensure that your brain has a steady supply of energy for hours. The walnuts and flaxseeds add an omega-3 fatty acid boost essential to great brain health.

MAKES 1 OR 2 SERVINGS

½ cup quick-cooking oatmeal, preferably gluten-free

½ cup water

½ apple

1 tablespoon ground flaxseeds

¼ teaspoon ground cinnamon

1 tablespoon unsalted raw walnuts

In a heat-safe bowl, place the oatmeal. In the microwave oven or on the stove top, bring the water to a boil. Cover the oatmeal with the boiling water. Let sit for 2 minutes while you finely chop the apple.

Add the apple, flaxseeds, cinnamon, and walnuts to the oatmeal. Stir until combined.

Serve immediately.

GLUTEN-FREE TOAST WITH COCO-ALMOND BUTTER AND PEACHES

Select a whole grain version of gluten-free bread, rather than the white rice or potato flour versions. A whole grain version is usually made with any combination of millet, amaranth, lima bean, navy bean, or chickpea flour with some tapioca or arrowroot added for a soft texture. It should be available at most health food stores.

MAKES 2 SERVINGS

4 slices whole grain,
gluten-free bread

Coco-Almond Butter
(page 218)

1 fresh peach or about 1 cup
frozen peaches, thawed

Toast the bread. Spread the toast with the Coco-Almond Butter and top it with the peach slices. Enjoy immediately.

COCO-ALMOND BUTTER

Coco-Almond Butter is an excellent source of brain-boosting medium-chain triglycerides and omega-3 fatty acids, as well as fiber, calcium, and magnesium. It's simple to make and a delicious addition to toast, sandwiches, celery sticks, or crackers.

MAKES ABOUT 3½ CUPS

3 cups unsalted raw almonds

⅓ cup coconut oil

½ cup flaxseed oil

In a food processor, pulse the almonds until finely ground.

Add the coconut and flaxseed oils. Pulse until smooth.

Store in a glass jar in the refrigerator for up to 2 weeks.

QUICK SPELT BREAD

While not gluten-free, spelt is an ancient wheat grain that many people tolerate well. This bread doesn't require any kneading or bread machines. You can throw it together in under 10 minutes, but you'll need to let it bake for 50 to 55 minutes.

MAKES 10 TO 12 SERVINGS

1¾ cups whole grain spelt flour

½ cup multigrain cereal or whole oats

1½ teaspoons aluminum-free baking powder

2 tablespoons water

1¼ cups rice milk or almond milk

2 tablespoons honey

½ cup extra-virgin olive oil or coconut oil

2 tablespoons ground flaxseeds (you can grind your own in a coffee grinder)

Preheat the oven to 350°F. Grease a 9" x 5" loaf pan.

In a food processor, pulse the flour, cereal or oats, and baking powder.

In a separate bowl, whisk together the water, milk, honey, oil, and flaxseeds. Slowly pour the flaxseed mixture into the flour mixture. Stir until well mixed.

Pour the batter into the loaf pan and bake for 50 to 55 minutes.

Let the bread cool in the pan on a rack for 5 to 10 minutes before removing it and serving it.

Beverages

GINGER LEMONADE

This refreshing lemonade with a kick is a great way to enjoy summer and boost your brain health at the same time. It offers ginger's potent anti-inflammatory compounds, known as gingerols, which are as delicious as they are healing. Thanks to the addition of stevia—a naturally sweet herb—this lemonade won't cause the typical blood sugar fluctuations common with sweetened and commercial versions of lemonade.

MAKES 4 SERVINGS

5 lemons

1 piece (3") fresh ginger

1½ teaspoons liquid stevia (about 90 drops), or to taste

6 cups water

Ice cubes

1 sprig fresh mint (optional)

Juice the lemons using a ceramic or wooden reamer (or an electric citrus juicer if you have one). Pour the juice into a large pitcher. Juice the ginger and add the juice to the pitcher. Add the stevia and pour in the water. Stir to mix.

Pour over ice and add the mint sprig, if using, to garnish.

ICED POMEGRANATE GREEN TEA

Reap the brain-boosting benefits of pomegranate juice and green tea all in one refreshing beverage.

MAKES 2 TO 4 SERVINGS

1 quart pure water

6 green tea bags

1 cup pomegranate juice

2 cups ice + additional,
   for serving

Stevia to taste (optional)

1 sprig fresh mint (optional)

In a kettle, bring the water to a boil. Pour into a teapot. Add the tea bags and let steep for 5 to 10 minutes. Allow the tea to cool.

In a large pitcher, pour the pomegranate juice and add the cooled tea. Add the 2 cups of ice and the stevia, if using. Stir until well mixed and garnish with the mint, if desired. Enjoy served over additional ice.

POMEGRANATE LEMONADE

Sipping this delicious lemonade is a great way to escape the stresses of modern life. And it's packed with brain-boosting nutrients from the pomegranate and lemon juice. Unlike most sweetened lemonade, thanks to the naturally sweet herb stevia, this lemonade keeps blood sugar levels stable, a key factor in providing a continual supply of energy to the brain and preventing brain-damaging inflammation. Plus it just tastes delicious.

MAKES 4 SERVINGS

5 lemons

1½ teaspoons liquid stevia (approximately 90 drops), or to taste

5 cups pure water

1 cup pomegranate juice

Ice cubes, for serving

Juice the lemons using a wooden or ceramic reamer (or an electric citrus juicer if you have one). Pour the juice into a large pitcher.

Add the stevia and pour in the water and pomegranate juice. Stir until well mixed.

Pour over the ice cubes and serve.

ALMOND MILK

Make your own fresh and creamy almond milk to drink on its own, use in baking, or use as a base in fruit smoothies.

MAKES 2 TO 4 SERVINGS

2 cups purified alkaline water

½ cup unsalted raw almonds

8 drops liquid stevia, or to taste

In a blender, pour the water. Add the almonds and stevia. Blend until smooth. Strain through cheesecloth or an almond milk–straining bag (available in most health food stores). Store in the refrigerator in a covered pitcher for up to 1 week.

SUPER-HEALTH-BOOSTING PUMPKIN SPICE "LATTE"

This recipe can be made with your favorite coffee, but I urge you to at least try it with roasted dandelion root. When dandelion root is roasted, it takes on a coffee-like flavor. You may be scoffing at the thought of a dandelion latte, but roasted dandelion root is perhaps the most overlooked natural superfood available. It grows almost everywhere and so is a renewable resource, to say the least.

If the thought of pulling up dandelions from your yard doesn't sound appealing, you can purchase dandelion root in most health food stores. It is available roasted or raw. If you're using raw dandelion, cut it into small chunks and place it on a baking sheet. Roast in a 200°F oven for 1 to 2 hours, depending on preference. (Longer roasting times produce a darker-roast taste.) Grind in a high-powered blender or coffee grinder. Store in an airtight glass jar. Some health food stores sell already roasted and ground dandelion root, often labeled "coffee substitute." If you're harvesting dandelion root yourself, be sure to choose an area free of pesticides and lawn sprays. I've found it easiest to harvest after a rainfall when the ground is soft.

This delicious pumpkin spice latte is devoid of the artificial ingredients that plague commercial varieties of the beverage and much lower in sugar. I tend to prefer a sweeter drink, so I simply increase the amount of coconut sugar used. You can serve this latte hot or iced, depending on your preference.

MAKES 2 SERVINGS

- 1½ cups almond or coconut milk
- ⅓ cup pumpkin puree
- 1 tablespoon roasted and ground dandelion root
- 1½ tablespoons coconut sugar, or to taste
- 1 teaspoon ground cinnamon + additional for sprinkling on top
- ⅛ teaspoon ground cloves
- ⅓ teaspoon ground nutmeg + additional for sprinkling on top

In a blender, combine the almond or coconut milk, pumpkin, dandelion root, sugar, 1 teaspoon cinnamon, cloves, and ⅓ teaspoon nutmeg. Blend until smooth and creamy. Sprinkle with additional cinnamon and nutmeg and serve.

To serve hot, pour the latte into a small saucepan. Set it over medium-high heat and, stirring occasionally, heat for 5 to 10 minutes, or until the desired temperature has been reached. Sprinkle with additional cinnamon and nutmeg and serve immediately.

WATER-BERRY JUICE

This juice is packed with important brain-boosting nutrients like glutathione, which helps to eliminate toxins from the body before they can access or damage the brain. But you'll love this juice for more than the health benefits.

MAKES 2 SERVINGS

2 cups cubed watermelon

1 cup frozen strawberries

In a blender, place the watermelon and the strawberries. Blend until smooth. Serve immediately.

GREEN GODDESS JUICE

The tart and slightly sweet Granny Smith apple adds punch to the nutrient-packed celery and cucumber, making this lovely light green juice both yummy and healthy. The mint adds the great, refreshing taste of summer, perfect for hot days.

MAKES 1 TO 2 SERVINGS

1 piece (4") cucumber

6 leaves mint

1 Granny Smith apple

3 ribs celery

In a juicer, combine the cucumber, mint, apple, and celery. Juice until well mixed. Serve immediately.

Appetizers, Dips, and Spreads

SOUTHWESTERN BRUSCHETTA

Here's my Mexican twist on an Italian favorite. I could eat this almost daily—it's that good. And it's easy to prepare for a snack, appetizer, or quick lunch.

MAKES 2 TO 4 SERVINGS

4–6 slices sprouted grain bread or yeast-free spelt or brown rice bread

1 clove garlic

Avo-Salsa (page 231)

Toast the bread until fairly crisp.

Rub each slice of toast with the garlic.

Place the toast on serving dishes and top it with the Avo-Salsa. Serve immediately.

GUACAMOLE

Serve this dip with tortilla chips or carrot sticks, celery sticks, sliced red or green bell peppers, and broccoli or cauliflower florets. Or use it as a spread on wraps and sandwiches. Eat it soon after making it, or the guacamole will discolor.

MAKES 2 TO 4 SERVINGS

1 avocado, peeled and pitted

Juice of ½ lime

1 tablespoon organic cold-pressed flaxseed oil

Pinch of Celtic sea salt

In a food processor, place the avocado, lime juice, oil, and salt. Puree until smooth. (Or use a hand blender.)

Garlic Guacamole

Add 1 clove of freshly minced garlic with the avocado.

BRAIN-BOOSTING BUTTER

Serve this soft, healthier butter substitute on warm bread, toast, steamed or roasted vegetables, or any of your favorite foods. Don't use it for cooking, as the omega-3 fatty acids found in flaxseed oil are volatile when heated.

MAKES ABOUT 1 CUP

½ cup organic extra-virgin coconut oil

½ cup organic cold-pressed flaxseed oil

In a small saucepan over low heat, liquefy the coconut oil. Immediately remove the pan from the heat and add the flaxseed oil, stirring until well mixed. Pour into a serving container and refrigerate until firm.

Store in an airtight container in the refrigerator for up to 6 months.

Michelle's Better Basil Butter

Immediately after adding the flaxseed oil, stir in a handful of chopped fresh basil.

BRAIN-BUILDING SALSA

In only 5 to 10 minutes, you can enjoy this incredible fresh salsa, and it's so versatile! There are so many delicious uses for this yummy salsa. Serve it with baked tortilla chips or bean chips (available in most health food stores), on celery sticks, on top of a plate of greens in place of dressing, or on toasted bread for a quick and delicious appetizer.

MAKES 4 TO 6 SERVINGS

1 clove garlic

½–1 small chile pepper, stem and seeds removed (wear plastic gloves when handling)

1 scallion, cut into 2" pieces

Small handful of fresh cilantro

3 large tomatoes, quartered

Juice of 1 lime

2 teaspoons ground psyllium husks

½ teaspoon unrefined sea salt

In a food processor, place the garlic and chile pepper. Process until finely minced.

Add the scallion, cilantro, tomatoes, lime juice, psyllium husks, and salt. Pulse until coarsely chopped.

Store in an airtight container in the refrigerator for up to 3 days.

Avo-Salsa

Add peeled, pitted, and cubed avocado just prior to serving. Toss gently to combine. The avocado cuts some of the heat and adds a creamy texture to the salsa.

POMEGRANATE SALSA

Use this pomegranate salsa as a refreshing topping for chicken or salmon. As an attractive appetizer, it's also delicious spooned into endive cups.

MAKES 8 SERVINGS

1 pomegranate

1 red onion, finely chopped

1–2 jalapeño chile peppers, finely chopped (wear plastic gloves when handling)

Juice of 2 limes

¼ teaspoon unrefined sea salt

Cut the pomegranate in half. Working over a fine sieve set over a bowl, use your fingers or a small spoon to extract the pulp-encased seeds from the light-colored membrane. Allow any juice to fall into the bowl. Add the seeds (discarding the membrane), onion, 1 or 2 peppers (depending upon desired heat), lime juice, and salt. Stir to mix. Cover and refrigerate for several hours before serving.

HUMMUS

Hummus is a delicious Middle Eastern dip that has been part of that culture for thousands of years. It adds important fiber, vitamin C, iron, and calcium to your diet. Serve it on sandwiches, as a dip for crudités, on wraps, or with bean tortilla chips (available in most health food stores). I love it scooped up with celery as an appetizer or alongside a meal.

MAKES 4 SERVINGS

2 cups cooked chickpeas

Juice of 1 lemon

1 large or 2 small cloves garlic

¼ cup raw tahini (also known as sesame butter)

In a food processor, combine the chickpeas, lemon juice, garlic, and tahini. Puree until smooth.

Store in an airtight container in the refrigerator for up to 1 week.

Soups and Stews

VEGGIE AND WILD RICE SOUP

This delicious and hearty soup is wonderful on a cool evening. Thanks to the wild rice and all of the vegetables, it is packed with nutrition.

MAKES 6 TO 8 SERVINGS

2 medium onions, finely chopped

3 tablespoons olive oil

2 carrots, chopped

2 potatoes, chopped

1 small sweet potato, chopped

½ small butternut squash, chopped

½ cup wild rice

2 teaspoons unrefined sea salt

10 cups water

1 teaspoon dried basil

Dash of ground red pepper

In a large pot over medium-low heat, cook the onions in the oil, stirring frequently, for 10 minutes or until lightly browned.

Add the carrots, potatoes, sweet potato, squash, rice, salt, water, basil, and red pepper. Turn the heat to high and bring the soup to a boil. Reduce the heat to low and let simmer for 1 hour.

Alternatively, you can combine the cooked onions with the carrots, potatoes, sweet potato, squash, rice, salt, water, basil, and red pepper in a slow cooker. Cook on high for 6 to 8 hours.

RED LENTIL AND RICE SOUP

Red lentils are smaller than brown lentils and cook more quickly. This mildly spiced soup is brightened with fresh ginger. To add more heat, drizzle Asian chili oil in place of the olive oil.

MAKES 6 SERVINGS

- 2 tablespoons extra-virgin olive oil, plus more for drizzling
- 1 cup chopped onion
- 2 cloves garlic, chopped
- 2 carrots, chopped
- 1 tablespoon grated fresh ginger
- 2 teaspoons ground cumin
- 1½ cups dried red lentils
- 7 cups water
- 1 cup drained diced canned tomatoes or chopped fresh cherry tomatoes
- 1½ cups cooked brown rice
- Kosher salt and freshly ground black pepper

In a large, heavy saucepan over medium heat, heat the oil. Cook the onion for 5 minutes, or until soft. Add the garlic, carrots, ginger, and cumin and cook for 2 minutes. Add the lentils and water. Bring to a boil. Reduce the heat and simmer until the lentils are just tender, about 20 minutes. Add the tomatoes and rice and simmer for 5 minutes. Remove about a quarter of the soup (about 2 cups) and puree in a blender. Return to the saucepan and stir. Season to taste with salt and pepper. Drizzle with a little oil before serving.

ROASTED CARROT SOUP

This creamy soup is rich and delicious and takes minimal preparation time. I make it whenever I am not in the mood for cooking, since it is so easy. Just because it is easy doesn't mean it is short on flavor.

MAKES 2 TO 4 SERVINGS

6 large carrots, chopped

2 tablespoons extra-virgin olive oil

2 cloves garlic

½ teaspoon ground cumin

1 teaspoon unrefined sea salt

Dash of ground red pepper

3–4 cups water, depending on desired thickness

In a large pot over medium-low heat, cook the carrots in the oil, stirring frequently, for 20 to 30 minutes or until softened.

Add the garlic and continue cooking, stirring frequently, until the garlic is soft and the carrots are lightly browned.

In a blender, place the cooked carrots and garlic, cumin, salt, red pepper, and water. Blend until smooth.

Return the soup to the pot and heat through. If using a Vitamix blender, continue blending until the soup is hot, then serve immediately.

SAVORY LENTIL STEW

This hearty stew is perfect on a cold winter's night but is so delicious you'll want to eat it year-round. It's packed with thiamin, potassium, iron, molybdenum, and other minerals. At 26 percent, lentils have one of the highest levels of protein in plant-based foods. What's more, only 1 cup of cooked lentils provides almost 90 percent of your daily requirement for folate and over 15 grams of fiber (that's a lot!). I've tried making this stew with French, green, and orange lentils—all with successful results—so use whatever kind you have on hand. And there's no need to worry about cooking them in advance. All you need are dried lentils. Enjoy.

MAKES 4 TO 6 SERVINGS

1 tablespoon extra-virgin olive oil

1 medium onion, finely chopped

1½ cups dried lentils

8 cups water

1 medium sweet potato, finely chopped

1 medium potato, finely chopped

2 ribs celery, chopped

1 teaspoon dried basil

1 teaspoon dried oregano

½ teaspoon dried thyme

1 teaspoon celery seeds

1½ teaspoons unrefined sea salt

Freshly ground black pepper to taste

In a large pot over medium heat, heat the oil. Add the onion and cook, stirring frequently, until lightly browned.

Add the lentils, water, sweet potato, potato, celery, basil, oregano, thyme, celery seeds, salt, and pepper. Turn the heat to high and bring to a boil. Cover and simmer over medium-low heat for 1 hour, or until the lentils are cooked.

Alternatively, as a simple time-saver, combine all the ingredients in a slow cooker in the morning. Cook on low heat for 6 to 8 hours. This delicious and hearty stew will be ready by the time you get home from work!

CHICKEN PHO WITH BUCKWHEAT NOODLES

Bok choy is a Chinese cabbage that has a sweet flavor and is packed with beta-carotene, vitamin C, and calcium. It is delicious in this classic Asian one-dish soup.

MAKES 4 SERVINGS

- 4 ounces low-sodium buckwheat (soba) noodles
- 2 teaspoons toasted sesame oil, divided
- 12 ounces chicken tenders, cut into thin strips
- 4 cups low-sodium organic chicken broth
- 8 baby bok choy, quartered lengthwise
- ½ cup shelled edamame
- ½ red bell pepper, cut into thin strips
- 1 small bunch scallions, sliced
- 1 teaspoon reduced-sodium soy sauce
- ½ cup cilantro, coarsely chopped
- Lime wedges, for serving

Prepare the noodles according to package directions, cooking about 1 minute less than directed (about 4 minutes). Drain well. Meanwhile, in a large soup pot over medium-high heat, heat 1 teaspoon of the sesame oil. Cook the chicken for 4 minutes, stirring, or until browned. Add the broth and bring to a gentle boil. Add the bok choy and edamame, reduce the heat, and simmer for 4 minutes, or until the chicken is cooked through and the vegetables are tender. Stir in the pepper and scallions. Cook for 2 minutes. Remove from the heat and stir in the remaining 1 teaspoon sesame oil, the soy sauce, and cilantro. Divide the noodles and soup among 4 bowls. Serve with lime wedges.

MISO SOUP

This is the simplest soup I've ever made. Plus, it's warm and delicious, particularly on a cold winter evening. You can even enjoy this soup as a Japanese-style breakfast. It's a great way to get more micro-mineral-packed seaweed into your diet.

MAKES 2 SERVINGS

3 cups water

3 teaspoons miso

1 scallion, green part only, chopped

2 tablespoons chopped (½") silken tofu

1 tablespoon arame or dulse seaweed, cut into thin strips (optional)

In a medium pot over medium-high heat, heat the water until boiling. Remove the pot from the heat.

Add the miso and whisk until well blended.

Add the scallion, tofu, and seaweed (if using). Let sit for a few minutes until the seaweed is soft. Stir and serve.

SLOW-COOKER SPLIT PEA SOUP

Like all members of the legume family, split peas are loaded with fiber—you'll enjoy 14 grams of fiber in this soup from the split peas alone! Be sure to drink plenty of water to help the fiber do its job of eliminating toxins that can interfere with brain health.

MAKES 8 SERVINGS

1 pound dried split green peas

3 ribs celery, chopped

2 cloves garlic, minced

1 large yellow onion, chopped

3 carrots, chopped

½ cup chopped fresh parsley

2 teaspoons herbes de Provence, 1 tablespoon dried thyme, or 1 tablespoon curry powder

2 bay leaves

1 teaspoon unrefined sea salt

Freshly ground black pepper

8 cups water

In a slow cooker, combine the peas, celery, garlic, onion, carrots, parsley, herbs, bay leaves, salt, pepper, and water. Cook on low for 8 to 9 hours or on high for 4 to 5 hours, or until the peas are completely cooked and softened. Adjust the seasonings and remove the bay leaves before serving.

HEARTY CHICKPEA SOUP

The spicy, pungent mix of cinnamon and ginger is a warming backdrop for this healthy, colorful soup.

MAKES 4 SERVINGS

2 tablespoons olive oil

1 rib celery, finely chopped

1 carrot, chopped

1 onion, chopped

2 teaspoons minced garlic

1 teaspoon ground cinnamon

¼ teaspoon ground turmeric

¼ teaspoon ground ginger or grated fresh ginger

Pinch of saffron (optional)

2 cups water

1 can (15 ounces) chickpeas, rinsed and drained

1 can (14½ ounces) diced or stewed tomatoes with no salt added

2 cups baby spinach leaves

Lemon wedges (optional)

In a medium saucepan over medium heat, heat the oil. Cook the celery, carrot, onion, and garlic, stirring occasionally, for 3 to 5 minutes, or until starting to soften. Add the cinnamon, turmeric, ginger, and saffron, if desired. Cook for 1 to 2 minutes, or until the spices are fragrant. Add the water, chickpeas, and tomatoes (with juice). Bring to a boil. Reduce the heat to a simmer. Cook, partially covered, for 25 minutes, or until the vegetables are tender. Stir in the spinach and cook for 2 minutes, or until wilted. Garnish with the lemon wedges, if desired.

CURRIED SWEET POTATO AND APPLE SOUP

This fall-inspired soup combines a number of potent brain-boosting foods. You'll benefit from the curcumin in the curry powder, the fiber in the sweet potatoes, and the antioxidants in the apples, but most of all, you'll probably be struck by its smooth and creamy texture—perfect for a brisk autumn day.

MAKES 8 SERVINGS

1 tablespoon olive oil

1 large onion, sliced

2 cloves garlic, sliced

1 tablespoon grated fresh ginger

1 teaspoon curry powder

¾ teaspoon ground cumin

½ teaspoon unrefined salt

¼ teaspoon ground cinnamon

4 cups water

1¼ pounds sweet potatoes, peeled and cut into chunks

3 large Granny Smith apples, peeled, cored, and cut into chunks

½ cup chopped cilantro

In a large saucepan or Dutch oven over medium heat, heat the oil. Cook the onion and garlic, stirring occasionally, for 5 minutes, or until tender. Add the ginger, curry powder, cumin, salt, and cinnamon. Cook, stirring constantly, for 1 minute. Add the water, sweet potatoes, and apples and bring to a boil over high heat. Reduce the heat to low, cover, and simmer, stirring often, for 20 minutes, or until the sweet potatoes are very tender. In a food processor or blender, puree the soup in batches until very smooth. Reheat if necessary. Stir in the cilantro.

Salads and Salad Dressings

Tossing Around Salad Ideas

If you avoid salads at any cost, thinking they consist only of iceberg lettuce and a couple slices of starchy tomato topped with some chemical- and sugar-laden bottled dressing, you will be happy to learn that brain-boosting salads are so much better than that. These excellent salads can be gourmet meals in themselves. I encourage you to make at least one large green salad part of your daily plan. Once you get started with this new habit, you'll see how easy and enjoyable—and creative—it can be. I compiled the following list of ingredients to make it easy for you to throw together delicious, nutritious salads. Remember: This list is just a starting point. You can use many other possible ingredients to vary your salads from day to day.

CREATE A GOURMET BRAIN-BOOSTING SALAD IN MINUTES

Alfalfa sprouts

Almonds, slivered or chopped

Apples, sliced or grated

Apricots, dried or fresh, chopped

Avocado

Basil, chopped

Beetroot, grated

Bell peppers (green, yellow, or red)

Blackberries

Blueberries

Boston lettuce

Broccoli, chopped

Broccoli sprouts

Brown rice, cooked

Cabbage, grated

Carrots, julienned or grated

Celeriac (celery root)

Celery

Cherries, pitted

Chickpeas

Cilantro (coriander), chopped

Clover sprouts

Cucumber

Edible flowers

Endive

Fenugreek sprouts

Flaxseeds, ground

Gingerroot, freshly grated

Grapefruit slices

Grapes (preferably purple or red)

Great Northern beans

Hazelnuts, chopped

Kidney beans

Leaf lettuce

Legumes of any type

Lima beans

Mint, chopped

Mixed greens (mesclun)

Mung bean sprouts

Mushrooms, raw or cooked

Olives

Onion sprouts

Orange slices

Parsley, chopped

Peaches, sliced

Pea shoots

Peas, fresh

Pine nuts

Pinto beans

Plums

Pomegranate seeds

Pumpkin seeds

Radicchio

Radishes

Raspberries

Red clover sprouts

Romaine lettuce

Rosemary, freshly chopped

Sage, freshly chopped or cooked
  in a little olive oil until crispy

Scallions

Sesame seeds

Spinach

Strawberries

Sunflower seeds

Sweet potato, grated

Tomatoes

Walnuts, raw, unsalted

Watercress

Wild rice, cooked

Wild salmon, smoked or cooked

I'll often sauté or roast a few of my favorite foods, like sweet potato wedges, red bell pepper slices, or onions, and top a large plate of greens and raw veggies with them. Toss with one of my favorite dressings (see opposite page), and you have an instant and delicious gourmet salad. The warmth of these cooked ingredients offers a nice contrast with the crunchy colder salad ingredients, particularly in the winter months.

Vegetable Crudités

You can add crunchy vegetables or fruit slices to a salad, or you can eat them on their own or with a delicious dip. I try to keep a container packed with veggies that I've sliced or chopped into finger food for those days when I'm less than enthusiastic about preparing dinner or snacks. Many veggies are perfect for this purpose, including carrots or baby carrots, turnips, cucumbers, celery, radishes, green beans, cauliflower, tomato wedges, broccoli, and red, green, and yellow bell peppers. If you want to add fruit, good options include apples, pineapple, tangerine, oranges, and pears. But you're really only limited by availability.

Salad Dressings

Don't be intimidated by the thought of making your own salad dressings. They take only a couple of minutes, can be made in advance and stored in the refrigerator, and are so much healthier than store-bought dressings.

Dressings can be made from cold-pressed oils such as extra-virgin olive oil, walnut oil, flaxseed oil, or a blend of healthy oils like Udo's Blend (available in most health food stores). You can add freshly squeezed lemon or lime juice, apple cider vinegar (make sure it has a live culture in it, which means there will be some sediment in the bottom of the bottle), balsamic vinegar, or red or white wine vinegar (free of added sulfites). You will find some excellent salad dressings in the following recipes.

Typically, the ratio of acid (lemon or vinegar) to oil is 1:3, making it easy to whip up your own creations. Then just add herbs, berries, or other ingredients to give your dressing even more flavor and nutrients. Shake all the ingredients together in a covered jar or use a hand blender or personal blender to blend them together for a thicker, smoother dressing. Most dressings will keep for about a week in the fridge. I suggest keeping two or three on hand to add variety to your salads when you're pressed for time.

WARM BLACK BEAN SALAD

If you're looking for something different from the typical green salad, this delicious salad delivers. And it is perfect during colder weather when it can be hard to get excited about cold salads. This one is warm, hearty, and delicious.

MAKES 2 TO 4 SERVINGS

1 medium onion, finely chopped

1 tablespoon extra-virgin olive oil

1 can (15 ounces) black beans, rinsed and drained

½ teaspoon dried oregano

½ teaspoon unrefined sea salt

1 tomato, chopped

Handful of fresh basil, finely chopped

In a medium skillet over medium heat, cook the onion in the oil, stirring frequently, for 10 minutes or until slightly browned. Add the beans, oregano, and salt and continue to cook, stirring frequently, for 1 to 2 minutes or until the beans are heated through.

Remove the skillet from the heat and stir in the tomato and basil. Serve immediately.

SALADE DE PROVENCE

This delightful salad incorporates the lovely fragrance of lavender in the herbes de Provence. The combination of blueberries with the lavender is splendid.

MAKES 4 SERVINGS

DRESSING

¼ cup balsamic vinegar

¾ cup extra-virgin olive oil

1 teaspoon honey

1 teaspoon herbes de Provence

Dash of Himalayan crystal salt or Celtic sea salt

Dash of freshly ground black pepper

SALAD

1 bag (5 ounces) mixed greens

Handful of alfalfa sprouts or clover sprouts

1 avocado, peeled, pitted, and sliced

1 cup fresh blueberries

To make the dressing: In a jar with a tight-fitting lid, place the vinegar, oil, honey, herbes de Provence, salt, and pepper. Cover and shake until well blended. (Alternatively, you may use a hand blender or personal blender.)

To make the salad: In a bowl, toss the mixed greens with the desired amount of dressing.

Place the dressed greens on serving plates. Top with the sprouts, avocado slices, and blueberries. Serve immediately.

MEDITERRANEAN BEAN, POTATO, AND VEGETABLE SALAD PLATTER

This hearty salad is perfect for a summer picnic, or any time you want to enjoy the lush, lemon-infused flavors of the Mediterranean.

MAKES 4 SERVINGS

2 cups canned kidney beans, rinsed and drained

3 small cooked red potatoes, sliced

½ cup balsamic vinegar

2 tablespoons minced garlic

2 tablespoons lemon juice

1 tablespoon honey

3 tablespoons olive oil

¼ cup finely chopped red onion

¼ teaspoon unrefined sea salt

3 cups torn leaf lettuce

½ cup sliced red bell pepper

½ cup sliced green bell pepper

1 large tomato, cut into wedges

Freshly ground black pepper

In a large bowl, combine the beans, potatoes, vinegar, garlic, lemon juice, honey, oil, onion, and salt. Stir gently. Let marinate at room temperature for 20 minutes. Line a platter with the lettuce; arrange the bell peppers and tomato around the edge. Strain the beans and potatoes from the marinade; pile in the center of the platter. Drizzle the marinade over the vegetables. Add black pepper to taste.

ROASTED SWEET POTATO SALAD

Roasting the sweet potatoes is an easy way to maximize their natural sweetness. When you're trying to make sure 80 percent of your diet is composed of fruits and vegetables, this recipe will help you hit the mark.

MAKES 4 SERVINGS

2 tablespoons olive oil

¼ teaspoon unrefined sea salt

¼ teaspoon freshly ground black pepper

2 pounds sweet potatoes, scrubbed and cut into 1" chunks

2 large red bell peppers, cut into 1" pieces

2 tablespoons white balsamic or white wine vinegar

1 pound spinach or arugula, torn into bite-size pieces

Preheat the oven to 425°F. In a large roasting pan, combine the oil, salt, and black pepper. Add the sweet potatoes and bell peppers and toss to coat well. Roast, shaking the pan occasionally, for 40 minutes, or until the potatoes are tender. Remove from the oven and stir in the vinegar. Place the spinach or arugula in a large serving bowl. Add the potato mixture and toss to coat well. Serve immediately.

CITRUS-GINGER SALAD

Don't let the strong-flavored ingredients fool you—this salad is amazing. It's one of my favorites. Even if I'm not in the mood for salad, I enjoy this one. It is packed with nutritious ingredients like greens, sprouts, garlic, ginger, and citrus fruit juice that give your body and brain a boost.

MAKES 2 TO 4 SERVINGS

SALAD

½ onion, finely sliced (almost like shavings)

Juice of ½ lemon or lime

Dash of unrefined sea salt

1 tablespoon olive oil

1 piece (2") fresh ginger, julienned

1 large or 2 small cloves garlic, julienned

1 package (5 ounces) mixed greens

1–2 large handfuls of mung bean sprouts

1 package (6 ounces) alfalfa sprouts, clover sprouts, or sprouts of your choice (about 2 cups if you grow your own)

DRESSING

Juice of ½ grapefruit

Juice of ½ lemon or lime

Juice of ½ orange or mandarin orange

Extra-virgin olive oil

Unrefined sea salt

Freshly ground black pepper

To make the salad: Place the onion slices in a small bowl. Add the lemon or lime juice and sprinkle the salt over. Set aside and let soak for at least 5 minutes. This mellows the flavor of the onion.

Heat the oil in a small skillet over low heat. Add the ginger and garlic and cook for 3 to 5 minutes, or until browned. Remove from the heat and reserve.

Place the mixed greens on serving plates as a salad base. Top with the mung bean sprouts, other sprouts of your choice, and the reserved onion slices. (Reserve the onion soaking liquid for the dressing.)

To make the dressing: In a jar with a tight-fitting lid, combine the grapefruit juice, lemon or lime juice, orange juice, oil, salt, pepper, and reserved soaking liquid from the onions. Shake until well mixed.

Pour the dressing over the salads. Top with the reserved garlic and ginger crisps. Serve immediately.

Citrus Sensation Salad

Add blood orange, orange, or grapefruit slices to the salad. Top with avocado slices.

THAI NOODLE SALAD

Don't be alarmed by the lengthy ingredients list. You can assemble this delicious and incredibly fresh-tasting salad in 10 minutes. And if you're missing a couple of the salad ingredients, don't worry—just use what you have. After creating it the first time, I ate it every day for a week. It's that good! As an added bonus, you can make the dressing ahead and store it in the fridge for a week for a quick and easy lunch or dinner.

MAKES 4 SERVINGS

SALAD

- 1 package (8 ounces) brown rice soba, udon, or spaghetti noodles
- ½ package (5 ounces) baby romaine lettuce leaves
- 2 cups mung bean sprouts
- 1 carrot, grated
- 1 red bell pepper, cut into 2" strips

- ½ cup snow peas, cut in half lengthwise (optional)
- 1 scallion, diagonally sliced
- ½ cup chopped fresh cilantro
- ½ cup unsalted raw peanuts
- Lime wedges, for garnish

DRESSING

- ¼ cup chopped fresh cilantro
- ¼ cup chopped fresh mint
- ½ scallion
- 1 clove garlic
- 1 piece (1") fresh ginger
- 2 tablespoons fresh lime juice

- 2 tablespoons extra-virgin olive oil
- ½ cup almond milk
- ¾ teaspoon salt
- Dash of ground red pepper

To make the salad: Cook the noodles according to package directions, drain, and set aside. While the noodles are cooking, make the dressing.

To make the dressing: In a wide-mouthed jar, place the cilantro, mint, scallion, garlic, ginger, lime juice, oil, almond milk, salt, and ground red pepper. Blend with a hand blender. (Alternatively, place all the ingredients in a small blender or food processor and blend until well mixed.)

Place a base of lettuce on each plate. Add a handful of noodles to each. Then top with plenty of mung bean sprouts, carrot, red bell peppers, and snow peas (if using). Drizzle with the dressing. Sprinkle the scallion, cilantro, and peanuts on top. Garnish with the lime wedges.

RICE SALAD WITH CURRIED TOFU

Opting for brown rice over white makes this dish a nutritional knockout. While both varieties contain an identical amount of carbs, brown rice contains four times as much insoluble fiber and magnesium.

MAKES 4 SERVINGS

1 package (15 ounces) extra-firm tofu

2 tablespoons olive oil, divided

1 teaspoon curry powder, divided

1 teaspoon unrefined sea salt, divided

⅓ cup shredded coconut

2 cups cooked brown rice

1 cup shelled edamame

¼ cup sunflower seeds

¼ cup pumpkin seeds

½ cup cherry tomatoes, halved

Freshly ground black pepper

Preheat the oven to 350°F. Cut the tofu into ½" cubes. Toss with 1 tablespoon of the oil, ½ teaspoon of the curry powder, ½ teaspoon of the salt, and the coconut. Arrange the tofu on a rimmed baking sheet and bake for 15 minutes. Meanwhile, in a large bowl, whisk the remaining 1 tablespoon olive oil, ½ teaspoon curry powder, and ½ teaspoon salt. Add the brown rice, edamame, sunflower seeds, pumpkin seeds, and tomatoes. Season to taste with pepper. Stir in the cooked tofu. Serve warm or at room temperature.

WILD RICE SALAD WITH CORN AND BEANS

This salad works well as either a main dish or a side accompaniment for chicken or fish. When fresh corn is in season, don't hesitate to use a few ears in place of the canned corn.

MAKES 6 SERVINGS

½ cup wild rice

1 can (11 ounces) low-sodium whole kernel corn, drained

1 can (14–19 ounces) black beans, rinsed and drained

2 scallions, chopped

½ small red bell pepper, chopped

1 small bunch cilantro, chopped

Juice of 1 lemon

¼ teaspoon unrefined sea salt

⅛ teaspoon freshly ground black pepper

Prepare the rice according to package directions. Meanwhile, in a serving bowl, combine the corn, beans, scallions, bell pepper, cilantro, lemon juice, salt, and black pepper. Add the rice and toss to combine. Serve warm or at room temperature.

QUINOA SALAD WITH CHERRIES AND PECANS

This sweet, nutty salad is loaded with protein from the quinoa and pecans. In fact, you might enjoy any leftovers for breakfast as a gluten-free alternative to breakfast cereal.

MAKES 4 SERVINGS

1½ cups water

1 cup quinoa, rinsed and drained

½ cup pecans

½ teaspoon olive oil

1 red onion, chopped

1 tablespoon honey

¼ teaspoon ground cinnamon

2 cups dark, sweet cherries, fresh or frozen

2 tablespoons chopped fresh parsley

In a medium saucepan, bring the water to a boil. Add the quinoa, cover, and reduce the heat to low. Simmer for 12 to 15 minutes, or until the water is absorbed. Uncover and allow to cool. Meanwhile, in a medium nonstick skillet over medium-high heat, cook the pecans, shaking the pan often, for 3 to 5 minutes, or until lightly toasted. Transfer to a plate to cool.

Heat the oil on medium-high in the same skillet. Cook the onion for 5 to 7 minutes, or until beginning to brown. Remove from the heat and stir in the honey and cinnamon. Set aside to cool. While the onion mixture and quinoa cool, pit the fresh cherries, if using, or thaw the frozen cherries in the microwave according to package directions. Coarsely chop the cherries. In a large bowl, combine the quinoa, cherries, onion mixture, and pecans. Toss well and sprinkle with the parsley before serving.

PROTEIN-RICH QUINOA SALAD

If you're a fan of Middle Eastern tabbouleh salad, this quinoa combination is a good gluten-free alternative to try.

MAKES 6 SERVINGS

1 cup quinoa

2 plum tomatoes, chopped

1 bunch fresh parsley, coarsely chopped

½ cucumber, peeled, seeded, and chopped

¼ cup finely chopped red onion

1 tablespoon extra-virgin olive oil

Juice of 2 Key limes (or juice of ½ lemon or lime)

Freshly ground black pepper

Prepare the quinoa according to package directions. Transfer to a large bowl and allow to cool for about 30 minutes. Add the tomatoes, parsley, cucumber, onion, oil, and lime juice. Mix gently to combine. Season to taste with pepper. This salad is best served cold or at room temperature.

BROCCOLI STEM, QUINOA, AND EDAMAME SALAD

This ingenious salad solves the age-old problem of what to do with leftover broccoli stems. Plus, it's elegant and colorful enough to present as a first course for a dinner party.

MAKES 4 SERVINGS

SALAD

- ¼ cup quinoa, rinsed well and drained
- 5 broccoli stems
- ¾ cup frozen, shelled edamame
- 1 small head radicchio, torn into bite-size pieces
- ½ cup pomegranate seeds, plus more for garnish (see note)

DRESSING

- 3 tablespoons extra-virgin olive oil
- 1 tablespoon rice wine vinegar
- 1 tablespoon finely chopped shallot
- 1 teaspoon grated fresh ginger
- ¼ teaspoon Dijon mustard
- ½ teaspoon unrefined sea salt, plus more to taste
- ⅛ teaspoon freshly ground black pepper, plus more to taste

To make the salad: Prepare the quinoa according to package directions. Allow to cool to room temperature. Meanwhile, use a vegetable peeler to remove the thick outer layer of each broccoli stem. When the soft inner flesh is revealed, use long, even strokes to shave off thin ribbons of broccoli. You should have 2½ to 3 cups of broccoli ribbons when you're done. Fill a large bowl with ice water to create an ice bath. Bring a medium saucepan of water to a boil. Place the stems and frozen edamame into the boiling water for 2 minutes, then drain and immediately transfer the vegetables to the ice bath. Drain and pat dry with a clean tea towel or paper towels.

To make the dressing: In a large mixing bowl, whisk together the oil, vinegar, shallot, ginger, mustard, salt, and pepper.

To the dressing, add the broccoli stems, edamame, cooked quinoa, radicchio, and pomegranate seeds. Toss well to combine. Taste and adjust the seasoning with additional salt and pepper, if desired. Divide evenly among 4 salad plates and garnish with additional pomegranate seeds, if desired. Serve immediately.

Note: To release the seeds from a fresh pomegranate, begin by cutting the fruit in half. Hold 1 half cut side down over a large mixing bowl and tap the outside of the fruit firmly with a wooden spoon. Repeat with the remaining half.

MEDITERRANEAN QUINOA SALAD

Grapes and pomegranate seeds provide a good dose of antioxidants, but in more practical terms, they also offer your tastebuds a wonderful sweet-and-sour contrast in this bright and crunchy salad.

MAKES 4 SERVINGS

½ cup quinoa

2 cups chopped romaine lettuce

10 red grapes, halved

½ cup pomegranate seeds (see note page 259)

1 tablespoon raw sunflower kernels

1 tablespoon extra-virgin olive oil

1 tablespoon pomegranate vinegar

3 tablespoons chopped fresh mint

3 tablespoons chopped fresh parsley

Freshly ground black pepper

Prepare the quinoa according to package directions. Transfer to a large bowl and allow to cool to room temperature. Add the lettuce, grapes, pomegranate seeds, and sunflower kernels. Toss gently to combine. In a small bowl, whisk the oil, vinegar, mint, and parsley until combined. Drizzle the dressing over the salad. Serve topped with a few grinds of fresh pepper.

MIXED GREENS SALAD WITH FALL FRUIT AND BEET DRESSING

This is a true fall salad; the dressing is homemade from beets and cranberry juice, and the salad includes pomegranate seeds, pear, and homemade croutons.

MAKES 4 SERVINGS

DRESSING

- 2 beets, cooked, peeled, and coarsely chopped
- 1 cup cranberry juice
- 3 tablespoons red wine vinegar
- 2 tablespoons Dijon mustard
- 2 tablespoons extra-virgin olive oil
- 1 shallot, chopped
- 1 clove garlic
  Dash of unrefined sea salt
  Dash of freshly ground black pepper

SALAD

- 8 cups mixed greens, torn into bite-size pieces
- 4 thick slices whole grain gluten-free bread, cubed and oven-toasted
- 1 large firm pear, cut into 16 wedges
- 1 Fuyu persimmon, chopped
  Seeds from 1 pomegranate (see note page 259)
- 2 tablespoons chopped toasted walnuts (see note)

To make the dressing: In a blender, combine the beets, cranberry juice, vinegar, mustard, oil, shallot, and garlic. Blend for 1 to 2 minutes, or until smooth. Season to taste with salt and pepper.

To make the salad: In a large bowl, toss the greens with the croutons and one-quarter of the dressing. Divide among 4 salad plates. Top with the pear wedges and persimmon. Drizzle with the remaining dressing. Sprinkle with the pomegranate seeds and walnuts.

Note: To toast the walnuts, place them in a dry nonstick skillet over medium heat. Toast the nuts, shaking the skillet often, for 3 to 5 minutes, or until fragrant.

BERRY SPECIAL CHICKEN SALAD

This salad comes together in minutes. If you'd like to prepare it ahead of time, prepare the dressing and salad ingredients separately and then toss everything together at the last minute.

MAKES 4 SERVINGS

¼ cup red wine or pomegranate vinegar

2 tablespoons extra-virgin olive oil

1 tablespoon unpasteurized honey

1 teaspoon poppy seeds

½ teaspoon dry mustard

6 cups rinsed, dried, and torn spinach leaves or 1 bag (6 ounces) baby spinach

2 cups chopped cooked organic chicken breast

2 cups sliced strawberries

1 cup pomegranate seeds (see note page 259)

In a large bowl, whisk together the vinegar, oil, honey, poppy seeds, and mustard. Add the spinach, chicken, strawberries, and pomegranate seeds. Toss to combine.

Entrées

LENTIL BURGERS

These lentil burgers are packed with flavor and a delicious alternative to meat burgers. Once you've tasted them, you'll want to make them a regular part of your diet.

MAKES 8

3 tablespoons extra-virgin olive oil, divided

1 medium onion, finely chopped

3 cups cooked lentils, drained and rinsed

1 cup quick-cooking oats

1 teaspoon unrefined sea salt

Pinch of ground black pepper

½ teaspoon ground cumin

2 tablespoons psyllium husks

Place 1 tablespoon of the oil in a skillet over medium-low heat. Add the onion and cook, stirring frequently, until lightly browned.

While the onion is cooking, mash the lentils in a large bowl using a potato masher. Add the oats, salt, pepper, cumin, and psyllium husks. Mash together until mixed.

Add the cooked onion to the lentil mixture and stir everything together.

Using your hands, form the mixture into burgers, being sure to press the burger ingredients together firmly.

Heat the remaining 2 tablespoons of oil in the skillet and cook the burgers for about 5 minutes per side, or until browned.

BASIL-LETTUCE-TOMATO-PEPPER (BLTP) SANDWICHES

A healthier take on the traditional BLT, this is one of my husband's all-time-favorite sandwiches. The basil, lettuce, tomato, and roasted red bell pepper are a fantastic flavor combination!

MAKES 2

4 slices whole grain gluten-free or ancient grain bread

2 tablespoons extra-virgin olive oil, divided

1 red bell pepper

1 package (1 ounce) fresh basil

6 whole peppercorns or freshly ground black pepper to taste

¼ teaspoon unrefined sea salt

1 clove garlic

1 tomato, sliced

Lettuce

Preheat the grill. Brush one side of each slice of bread with some of the olive oil.

Cut the bell pepper into 4 large pieces and brush with a small amount of the olive oil. Grill for 5 to 10 minutes, turning once. Remove from the grill.

In a mortar and pestle (or food processor, if you prefer) combine 1 tablespoon of the olive oil, the basil, peppercorns or ground black pepper, and salt until they form a fine paste.

Placing the oil-covered side down, grill the bread for 2 minutes and remove from the heat when finished.

Rub the clove of garlic over the grilled side of each slice of bread.

Spread the basil mix on the grilled side of 2 slices of bread.

Place the red pepper on top of the basil mix. Add the tomato and lettuce. Top with the other 2 slices of grilled bread and serve.

ROASTED HOISIN TOFU

Serve this tofu with brown rice as a meatless main course alongside a lightly dressed salad of napa cabbage or cucumbers. Or let it come to room temperature, refrigerate, and then cut into cubes to use in a salad, soup, stew, or stir-fry.

MAKES 4 SERVINGS

¼ cup hoisin sauce

2 tablespoons rice wine vinegar

1 tablespoon dark sesame oil

1 teaspoon Asian chili garlic sauce

2 packages (15 ounces each) extra-firm tofu, drained (see note)

Preheat the oven to 375°F. In a small bowl, stir together the hoisin, vinegar, sesame oil, and chili garlic sauce. Pat the tofu pieces dry and brush them all over with the hoisin mixture. Roast for 45 to 50 minutes, turning occasionally, or until browned and hot.

Note: To drain the excess water out of tofu, cut a block of tofu horizontally in half and then cut each piece crosswise in half to make rectangles roughly 3¼" x 2¼". Arrange the tofu pieces in an even layer on a baking sheet. Prop the baking sheet up at one end by at least 1" (more if possible) and have the other end overhang the sink. Cover with 2 thicknesses of paper towels and top with another baking sheet or a cutting board. Weight down with a heavy skillet or a few cans. Let the tofu drain into the sink for at least 30 minutes.

ROASTED MISO-GINGER TOFU

Use the roasted tofu in salads, cut up and added to stir-fries, or by itself as a meatless main course.

MAKES 4 SERVINGS

3 tablespoons miso paste

1 tablespoon olive oil

2 scallions, white and 2" of greens, thinly sliced

1 tablespoon grated fresh ginger

1 clove garlic, finely minced

2 packages (15 ounces each) extra-firm tofu, drained (see note page 265)

Preheat the oven to 375°F. In a small bowl, stir together the miso, oil, scallions, ginger, and garlic. Pat the tofu pieces dry and brush them all over with the miso mixture. Roast for 45 to 50 minutes, turning occasionally, or until browned and hot.

EASY TOFU STIR-FRY FOR ONE

Here's a simple weeknight meal for one that can help clear out small amounts of vegetables you might have lingering in the refrigerator. Simply multiply the recipe as necessary if you're feeding more than yourself. Throw in some leftover roasted tofu if you have it; add it to the stir-fry after the vegetables are cooked and before adding the sauce.

MAKES 1 SERVING

2 teaspoons coconut oil

4 ounces (about ¼ of 15-ounce package) extra-firm tofu, drained and cubed (see note page 265)

2 cloves garlic, minced

1 cup broccoli florets

¾ cup cauliflower, chopped

½ small carrot, sliced

2 scallions, sliced

2 tablespoons reduced-sodium stir-fry sauce

½ cup cooked brown rice

In a wok or large skillet over high heat, heat the oil. Cook the tofu, turning regularly, until it begins to brown, about 5 to 8 minutes. Add the garlic and cook until fragrant. Add the broccoli, cauliflower, and carrot and cook, covered, for 2 to 3 minutes, or until the vegetables begin to soften but still retain some crunch. Add the scallions and stir-fry sauce and toss to coat. Serve stir-fry over rice.

COCONUT CURRIED TOFU WITH MACADAMIA NUTS

Due to their high oil content, macadamia nuts should be stored in a cool, dry place and should be used within 4 weeks of opening. To extend their shelf life, keep them in your refrigerator or freezer.

MAKES 6 SERVINGS

1 cup brown basmati rice

1 tablespoon coconut oil

1 package (15 ounces) firm tofu, drained and cut into ¾" cubes (see note page 265)

½ teaspoon unrefined sea salt, divided

1 large onion, halved and thinly sliced

1 tablespoon red curry paste, plus more to taste

½ teaspoon curry powder

4 cups broccoli florets

1 cup light coconut milk

¾ cup reduced-sodium vegetable broth

1 cup frozen green peas

1 large tomato, cut into ¾" pieces

2 tablespoons lime juice

¾ cup chopped macadamia nuts

Prepare the rice according to package directions. In a large nonstick skillet over medium-high heat, heat the oil. Cook the tofu, turning once, for 6 to 8 minutes, or until golden brown. Sprinkle with ¼ teaspoon of the salt. With a slotted spoon, remove to a plate.

Add the onion to the skillet and cook, stirring frequently, for 3 to 4 minutes, or until browned. Stir in 1 tablespoon of the curry paste, the curry powder, and the remaining ¼ teaspoon salt. Taste and add more curry paste if desired. Add the broccoli, coconut milk, broth, and peas. Bring to a boil. Reduce the heat to low. Cover and simmer for 3 to 4 minutes, or until the broccoli is tender-crisp. Stir in the tomato, lime juice, and the reserved tofu. Simmer, stirring occasionally, for 2 to 3 minutes, or until the tofu is hot. Serve over the rice. Sprinkle with the macadamia nuts.

PINEAPPLE-BASIL RICE

I'm always trying to come up with unique and delicious ways to prepare brown rice to get more of this healthy grain (actually a seed) into my diet. It's so good, even brown rice haters will love it.

MAKES 2 TO 4 SERVINGS

1 cup brown rice

2 cups water

2 tablespoons coconut oil, divided

Large handful of fresh basil leaves

¾ cup finely chopped fresh pineapple

½ teaspoon unrefined sea salt

In a medium pot, combine the rice, water, and 1 tablespoon of the coconut oil. Bring to a boil over medium-high heat. Once the water begins to boil, immediately reduce the heat to low and let simmer, covered, for 45 to 50 minutes, or until all the water has been absorbed.

In a medium to large bowl, toss together the cooked rice, remaining 1 tablespoon of coconut oil, basil, pineapple, and salt until combined. Serve immediately.

CURRIED CHICKPEAS AND RICE

This delicious curry balances heat with sweetness. If you prefer, a more mild curry powder will yield a satisfying alternative. Just look for the signature yellow in your curry, which signifies the presence of turmeric, the powerful spice that can fight inflammation and plaque buildup in the brain.

MAKES 4 SERVINGS

1 cup instant brown rice

1 cup frozen peas

3 tablespoons olive oil

1 large onion, chopped

4 large cloves garlic, minced

½ teaspoon red-pepper flakes

2 teaspoons hot curry powder

1 tablespoon grated fresh ginger

¾ teaspoon unrefined sea salt

1 can (15 ounces) chickpeas, rinsed and drained

¼ cup golden raisins

¼ cup dark raisins

¾ cup light coconut milk

¼ cup lightly salted cashew halves

Prepare the rice according to package directions. Add the peas and remove from the heat. Cover and let stand for 10 minutes. Meanwhile, in a large skillet over medium heat, heat the oil. Cook the onion, garlic, and pepper flakes, stirring constantly, for 3 minutes, or until lightly browned. Add the curry powder, ginger, and salt. Cook for 1 minute, stirring constantly. Add the chickpeas, raisins, and coconut milk. Bring to a boil, reduce the heat to low, cover, and simmer, stirring occasionally, for 15 minutes, or until thickened. Transfer the rice to a serving bowl and top with the curry mixture. Sprinkle with the cashews.

GREEK QUINOA TOSS

If you toss this salad while it is still warm, the spinach will wilt and the tomatoes will soften considerably, yielding even more flavor to the finished dish.

MAKES 4 SERVINGS

1 cup frozen shelled edamame

¾ cup quinoa, rinsed

2 tablespoons fresh lemon juice

1 tablespoon olive oil

½ teaspoon dried oregano

¼ teaspoon unrefined sea salt

1 clove garlic, minced

3 cups baby spinach

1 cup grape tomatoes, halved

Prepare the edamame and quinoa according to package directions. In a large bowl, whisk together the lemon juice, oil, oregano, salt, and garlic. Add the spinach, tomatoes, edamame, and quinoa. Toss to coat well.

MILLET AND SWEET POTATO CAKES

Millet is a grain prized in Europe for its chewy texture. In this country, it's a frequent component in bird-seed mixtures. But don't let the birds get all its fiber and nutty flavor. Use it in recipes like this, where millet blends with a grated sweet potato in savory pancakes perfect for an evening meal.

MAKES 4 SERVINGS

1 cup vegetable broth

⅓ cup millet

1 small sweet potato, peeled and shredded

¼ cup finely chopped onion

2 organic eggs, lightly beaten

1 tablespoon almond flour

½ teaspoon dried thyme

⅛ teaspoon crushed red-pepper flakes

⅛ teaspoon unrefined sea salt

⅛ teaspoon freshly ground black pepper

1 tablespoon coconut oil

In a small saucepan, combine the broth and millet. Bring to a boil over medium-high heat. Reduce the heat to low, cover, and cook for 25 minutes, or until the millet is tender. Place in a medium bowl. Add the sweet potato, onion, eggs, flour, thyme, red-pepper flakes, salt, and black pepper. Mix well.

In a large skillet over medium-high heat, heat the oil. Drop spoonfuls of the batter into the skillet. Cook for 6 to 8 minutes, turning once, or until golden brown on both sides. Transfer to a plate and cover to keep warm. Repeat to use all of the batter.

Note: To freeze the cakes, place on a tray. Put in the freezer for 1 hour, or until solid. Stack, separated by small pieces of waxed paper, in a freezer-quality plastic bag. To use, thaw overnight in the refrigerator. Place in a 10" nonstick skillet, cover, and cook over low heat for 5 to 8 minutes, or until hot.

MOROCCAN STUFFED PEPPERS

These peppers are packed with brain-boosting ingredients, but it's likely the flavorful aroma of them baking is all that you'll need to convince you to make them a regular dish in your repertoire.

MAKES 4 SERVINGS

½ cup millet

4 small bell peppers, halved lengthwise (any colors, preferably a variety)

1½ cups vegetable broth, divided

1 tablespoon olive oil

1 small onion, chopped

1 can (15 ounces) chickpeas, rinsed and drained

2 cloves garlic, minced

1 teaspoon ground cumin

1 teaspoon curry powder

¼ teaspoon unrefined sea salt

4 cups coarsely chopped kale

1 small tomato, chopped

¼ cup finely chopped dried apricots

Prepare the millet according to package directions. Preheat the oven to 350°F. In a 13" x 9" baking dish, place the pepper halves cut sides down. Pour in ½ cup of the broth. Cover and microwave on high power for 10 minutes, or until the peppers soften. Turn the peppers over. Set aside.

In a large skillet over medium heat, heat the oil. Cook the onion and chickpeas for 8 minutes, stirring frequently. Add the garlic, cumin, curry powder, and salt. Cook, stirring, for 1 minute. Add the kale and remaining 1 cup broth. Increase the heat to high and bring to a boil. Reduce the heat to medium and simmer for 2 minutes, or until the kale is wilted. Stir in the millet, tomato, and apricots. Simmer for 2 minutes. Spoon the filling into the pepper halves. Bake for 25 to 30 minutes, or until the peppers are tender.

DAIRY-FREE PASTA ALFREDO WITH ASPARAGUS

This pasta is so rich and creamy that you won't miss the dairy products at all. The asparagus adds a delightful nuttiness that adds to the great flavor of the pasta.

MAKES 2 TO 4 SERVINGS

1 package (16 ounces) brown rice pasta

1 tablespoon extra-virgin olive oil

1 clove garlic, minced

1 tablespoon brown rice flour

1 cup unsweetened almond milk

½ teaspoon unrefined sea salt

Freshly ground black pepper to taste

1 bunch (about 1 pound) asparagus, cut into 1" pieces

In a large pot, cook the pasta according to package directions.

In the meantime, in a large pan over medium heat, heat the oil. Add the garlic and cook, stirring frequently, for 1 minute or until lightly golden. Add the rice flour and stir to combine, then cook for 30 seconds to 1 minute, or until lightly browned. Add the almond milk, salt, and pepper and stir for 1 to 2 minutes, or until combined and the mixture thickens. Add the asparagus pieces. Stir until the asparagus is cooked, about 5 to 10 minutes. Immediately stir the cooked pasta into the sauce. Toss and serve immediately.

GREEN BEAN RAGOUT

This Italian-inspired recipe is great as a side dish for pasta, chicken, fish, or your favorite Italian veggie dishes. It has a nutty flavor that complements the flavor of the tomato sauce.

MAKES 2 TO 4 SERVINGS

2 cloves garlic, minced or pressed

1 tablespoon extra-virgin olive oil

3 tomatoes, chopped

1½ cups fresh green beans, ends removed (if unavailable, use frozen)

1 small zucchini, cut into large chunks

⅛ teaspoon Himalayan crystal salt or Celtic sea salt, or to taste

Freshly ground black pepper to taste

In a medium saucepan over medium heat, cook the garlic in the oil, stirring frequently, for 1 to 2 minutes or until slightly golden.

Add the tomatoes, green beans, zucchini, salt, and pepper, and cover with a lid. Allow to simmer over medium-low heat for 10 to 15 minutes, or until the veggies are cooked but not mushy.

GREEN BEANS WITH WALNUTS

If you don't have walnut oil, use peanut oil or another tablespoon of olive oil.

MAKES 6 SERVINGS

1 pound green beans, trimmed and cut into 1" pieces

½ medium sweet onion, finely chopped

1 small clove garlic, minced

2 tablespoons olive oil

1 tablespoon walnut oil

1 tablespoon white wine vinegar

Unrefined sea salt

Freshly ground black pepper

¼ cup walnuts, toasted and chopped, for serving

In a steamer, cook the beans until tender-crisp, about 5 minutes. Transfer the hot beans to a serving bowl. Add the onion, garlic, olive oil, walnut oil, and vinegar. Season to taste with salt and pepper. Serve topped with the toasted walnuts.

STIR-FRIED ASPARAGUS WITH SESAME SEEDS

This quick stir-fry will probably come together faster than the local Chinese take-out place can have your order ready. Make sure to snap off the tough ends of the asparagus before cutting them. If the spears are especially thick, consider peeling the lower half.

MAKES 6 SERVINGS

4 teaspoons olive oil

½ cup thinly sliced scallions

2 teaspoons grated fresh ginger

1 teaspoon minced garlic

2½ pounds asparagus, cut into 2" pieces (about 5½ cups)

⅓ cup water

1 tablespoon sesame seeds, for serving

2 teaspoons dark sesame oil

¼ teaspoon unrefined sea salt

In a large skillet over medium-high heat, heat the olive oil. Cook the scallions, ginger, and garlic, stirring frequently, until fragrant, about 30 seconds. Add the asparagus and stir-fry until it turns bright green, about 1 minute. Add the water. Cover and steam until the asparagus is tender-crisp, 2 to 3 minutes.

Meanwhile, in a small skillet over medium heat, stir the sesame seeds until toasted, 2 to 4 minutes. Transfer to a plate. Add the sesame oil to the asparagus and stir-fry for 30 seconds. Remove from the heat, sprinkle with the salt, and toss to combine. Serve the asparagus sprinkled with the toasted sesame seeds.

CURRIED CAULIFLOWER

Cooking spices in a small amount of oil releases their aroma and flavor. To keep calories to a minimum, precook the cauliflower in water and then stir-fry with some oil, garlic, and curry powder. If you don't have parsley, substitute 1 tablespoon of minced scallion greens or 2 tablespoons of frozen baby peas. Toss with the cauliflower for about 1 minute, or until heated through.

MAKES 4 SERVINGS

1 small head cauliflower, cut into walnut-size florets

2 teaspoons olive oil

1 teaspoon minced garlic

½ teaspoon curry powder

¼ teaspoon unrefined sea salt

1 tablespoon finely chopped parsley (optional)

Freshly ground black pepper

Fill a large skillet with enough water to come ½" up the sides of the pan. Cover and bring to a boil over high heat. Add the cauliflower. Reduce the heat to medium-high, cover, and cook, stirring once, for 3 minutes, or until tender but still crisp. Tip the pan and spoon out most of the water into a measuring cup. Set aside.

Return the pan to the heat. Add the oil, garlic, curry powder, and salt. Cook, tossing frequently and adding a tablespoon at a time of the reserved water when the skillet appears dry. Scrape the bottom of the pan to release the flavorful browned bits. Cook for 5 minutes, or until the cauliflower is golden brown. Sprinkle with the parsley, if using. Season to taste with pepper.

GRILLED SALMON WITH PLUM-BLUEBERRY-GRAPE SALSA

I could eat this amazing dish regularly. The garam masala dry rub provides a wonderful contrast to the fresh, sweet taste of the fruit salsa. You'll enjoy the taste sensation, while your body will love the omega-3 fatty acids from the salmon and the disease-fighting proanthocyanidins found in the Plum-Blueberry-Grape Salsa.

MAKES 2 SERVINGS

SALMON

1 teaspoon garam masala powder

¼ teaspoon unrefined sea salt

2 salmon fillets or steaks

SALSA

1 black plum, pitted and chopped into small cubes

⅓ cup fresh or frozen blueberries

½ cup quartered purple grapes

Small handful of chopped fresh cilantro

Dash of Himalayan crystal salt or Celtic sea salt

Splash of white wine vinegar

½ teaspoon honey

To make the salmon: Preheat the grill. Rub the garam masala and salt into the top of the salmon fillets or steaks (the side without skin).

Grill for 3 minutes skin side down if using fillets or 5 minutes if using steaks. Turn and cook for 3 minutes if using fillets or 5 minutes if using steaks.

To make the salsa: In a small bowl, combine the plum, blueberries, grapes, cilantro, salt, vinegar, and honey. Toss to blend.

Spoon the salsa over the grilled salmon.

ROAST COD WITH POMEGRANATE-WALNUT SAUCE

The mild, clean flavor of cod is the perfect backdrop for the pomegranate and walnut combination in this dish. However, if cod is not available, haddock or flounder would make fine substitutions.

MAKES 4 SERVINGS

1 cup quinoa

1 tablespoon olive oil

1 shallot, finely chopped (about ¼ cup)

⅓ cup ground walnuts plus ¼ cup broken halves

3 cloves garlic, minced

⅓ cup dry red wine

¼ cup reduced-sodium vegetable broth

1½ tablespoons pomegranate molasses or frozen cranberry juice concentrate

1 tablespoon honey

4 cod fillets (6 ounces each)

Unrefined sea salt

Freshly ground black pepper

¼ cup chopped fresh parsley

Prepare the quinoa according to package directions. Meanwhile, in a medium skillet over medium heat, heat the oil. Cook the shallot, stirring, for 2 minutes, or until softened. Add the ground walnuts and garlic and cook, stirring, for 4 minutes, or until the walnuts are golden brown. Remove from the heat and add the wine, broth, molasses or juice, and honey. Return to the heat and simmer, stirring occasionally, for 4 minutes, or until thickened. Transfer the sauce to a gravy boat and set aside.

Heat the broiler. Season the fish with salt and pepper. Arrange in a single layer on a sheet pan lined with foil. Broil for 6 minutes, or until the fish flakes easily. Toss the quinoa with the parsley and broken walnuts. Spoon onto 4 plates and top with the fish and sauce.

ORANGE BALSAMIC HALIBUT WITH MINT AND DRIED CHERRIES

If you think you need to stick to salmon to reap the benefits of seafood, think again. A 6-ounce serving of halibut may help protect against Alzheimer's as it is an excellent source of niacin, providing more than half of the Daily Value.

MAKES 4 SERVINGS

1 cup brown basmati rice

2 tablespoons olive oil, divided

1 tablespoon chopped fresh mint, divided

1 small fennel bulb, thinly sliced

1 cup chopped onion

2 teaspoons minced garlic

Peel and juice from 1 medium orange

1 tablespoon balsamic vinegar

3 tablespoons dried cherries

2 cups chopped fresh or canned tomatoes (with juice)

½ teaspoon unrefined sea salt

¼ teaspoon freshly ground black pepper

4 skinless halibut steaks (about 1½ pounds)

Prepare the rice according to package directions. Toss with 1 tablespoon of the oil and 1 teaspoon of the mint. Cover and set aside.

In a large skillet over medium-high heat, heat the remaining 1 tablespoon oil. Cook the fennel, onion, and garlic, covered, for 4 to 6 minutes, stirring 2 or 3 times. Add the orange peel and juice, vinegar, cherries, tomatoes, and 1 teaspoon of the mint. Cover and cook for 4 to 6 minutes, or until the tomatoes begin to fall apart. Sprinkle the salt and pepper over the halibut. Bury the fish among the vegetables in the pan. Spoon some of the vegetables over the top of the fish. Cover the skillet, reduce the heat to medium low, and cook for 6 to 7 minutes, or until the fish is firm and flakes easily. Serve the fish over the rice and topped with the vegetables. Garnish with the remaining 1 teaspoon mint.

TOASTED MILLET SALAD WITH SALMON

Healthful omega-3 fatty acids are also found in other oily fish such as sardines and mackerel, so if you like, you can replace the salmon in this dish with one of these fish.

MAKES 4 SERVINGS

2½ cups + 2 tablespoons water, divided

1 teaspoon + 1 tablespoon olive oil, divided

1 cup millet

8 ounces boneless, skinless salmon fillets

1 teaspoon + 1 tablespoon reduced-sodium soy sauce, divided

2 cups snow peas, trimmed

¼ cup rice wine vinegar

1 tablespoon toasted sesame oil

2 teaspoons grated fresh ginger

1 teaspoon minced garlic

¼ teaspoon unrefined sea salt

½ cup finely sliced scallions

½ cup finely chopped red bell pepper

In a medium saucepan, bring 2½ cups of the water to a boil. Meanwhile, coat the bottom of a large skillet with 1 teaspoon of the olive oil. Add the millet and cook, stirring, over medium-low heat for 10 minutes, or until it gives off a toasted aroma. Add the boiling water to the skillet. Cover and cook for 25 minutes, or until the water is absorbed and the millet is tender. Uncover and allow to cool.

Meanwhile, coat the salmon with 1 teaspoon of the soy sauce. Set a large nonstick skillet over high heat for 1 minute. When hot, add the fish. Reduce the heat to medium and cook for 6 to 7 minutes, turning once, or until the fish is opaque. Remove from the heat and allow to cool in the pan. Break into 1" chunks.

Bring a small saucepan of water to a boil. Add the snow peas and cook for 1 minute. Drain, rinse, and then blot dry. Set aside. In a large bowl, whisk the vinegar, 2 tablespoons water, sesame oil, ginger, garlic, salt, and remaining 1 tablespoon olive oil and 1 tablespoon soy sauce. Reserve 1 tablespoon of the mixture. Toss the reserved millet with the dressing. In a small bowl, toss the scallions, pepper, reserved snow peas, and reserved dressing. Add half the vegetables and the salmon to the millet. Spoon the millet salad onto a platter. Top with the remaining vegetables.

SEARED SEA SCALLOPS WITH QUINOA PILAF

Here's a good recipe for special occasions because it is easy to make look as fancy as it is delicious. The saffron will render your quinoa a bright, beautiful yellow. Use ½ teaspoon of turmeric in its place if saffron isn't handy in your pantry.

MAKES 6 SERVINGS

SAUCE

2 cups pomegranate juice

1½ teaspoons reduced-sodium soy sauce

1½ teaspoons Chinese five-spice powder

¼ cup finely chopped shallot

2 teaspoons grated fresh ginger

PILAF

2 cups quinoa, rinsed very well

1 teaspoon olive oil

1 small onion, chopped

¼ teaspoon ground cinnamon

⅛ teaspoon saffron threads, crushed

⅛ teaspoon ground red pepper

½ cup raisins

½ cup dried cranberries

¼ cup toasted sliced almonds

2 teaspoons lemon juice

SCALLOPS

2 pounds large sea scallops, patted dry

Unrefined sea salt and freshly ground black pepper

2 tablespoons olive oil, divided

½ teaspoon sesame oil, divided

2 teaspoons black sesame seeds (optional)

To make the sauce: In a small pan over medium-low heat, combine the pomegranate juice, soy sauce, five-spice powder, shallot, and ginger and bring to a simmer. Simmer for 45 minutes, or until the sauce reduces to about ½ cup. Keep warm.

To make the pilaf: Meanwhile, prepare the quinoa according to package directions. When the quinoa is cooked, in a large skillet over medium-high heat, heat the oil. Cook the onion, stirring, for 5 minutes, or until translucent. Add the cinnamon, saffron, and red pepper and cook for 1 to 2 minutes, or until fragrant. Transfer the quinoa to the skillet and add the raisins, cranberries, almonds, and lemon juice. Toss to combine. Cover and set aside.

To make the scallops: Sprinkle the scallops with salt and black pepper to taste. In a large nonstick skillet over high heat, heat 1 tablespoon of the olive oil and ¼ teaspoon of the sesame oil. Cook half of the scallops for 4 minutes, turning once, or until opaque. Transfer to a plate and keep warm. Repeat with the remaining 1 tablespoon olive oil, ¼ teaspoon sesame oil, and scallops. Drizzle with the sauce and garnish with the sesame seeds, if using. Serve with the pilaf.

SHRIMP IN GREEN TEA-CURRY SAUCE

This dish is so simple to prepare, yet it's sophisticated enough to share with guests. The delicate tea flavor is delightfully enhanced by the subtle curry.

MAKES 6 SERVINGS

8 ounces brown rice pasta

1 cup boiling water

1 tablespoon green tea leaves

1 tablespoon coconut oil

1 pound large shrimp, peeled, deveined, and rinsed

¼ cup finely sliced scallions, white and light green parts, plus additional for garnish

2 teaspoons minced garlic

1½ teaspoons hot or mild curry powder

½ teaspoon unrefined sea salt

1 teaspoon toasted sesame oil

Chopped cilantro (if desired for garnish)

Prepare the pasta according to package directions, subtracting 2 minutes of the cooking time. Drain and return to the cooking pot to keep warm. In a heatproof container, combine the boiling water and tea leaves. Cover and steep for 5 minutes.

Meanwhile, in a large nonstick wok or skillet over high heat, heat the coconut oil. Cook the shrimp, scallions, garlic, curry powder, and salt, tossing, for 1 minute. Add the tea and half of the tea leaves. Cook for 1 minute, or until the shrimp are opaque. Use a slotted spoon to remove the shrimp to a plate and set aside.

Transfer the pasta to the wok or skillet. Reduce the heat to medium low. Cook, tossing, for 3 minutes, or until the pasta is al dente and the sauce has thickened. Return the shrimp to the pan. Drizzle with the sesame oil. Toss to combine. Garnish with the cilantro and additional scallions, if desired.

CHICKEN SUMMER ROLLS

If you'd like, use large, soft lettuce leaves in place of the rice wrappers. Set out bowls of the vegetables and have everyone make his or her own rolls.

MAKES 4 SERVINGS

SAUCE

⅓ cup low-sodium organic chicken broth

1 tablespoon reduced-sodium soy sauce

1 tablespoon fresh lime juice

1 teaspoon white wine vinegar

Pinch of ground red pepper

ROLLS

2 ounces low-sodium buckwheat noodles

8 round rice paper wrappers (8" diameter)

¼ cup chopped fresh mint leaves

¼ cup chopped cilantro

½ avocado, cut into 8 thin slices

1 cup fresh spinach, cut into strips

1 red bell pepper, cut into thin strips

1 carrot, shredded

1½ cups shredded cooked organic chicken breast

To make the sauce: In a medium bowl, whisk together the broth, soy sauce, lime juice, vinegar, and red pepper.

To make the rolls: Prepare the buckwheat noodles according to package directions, omitting the salt. Rinse under cold running water and drain well. Soak 1 rice paper wrapper in warm water for 30 to 60 seconds, or until soft. Carefully transfer to a clean work surface, preferably a wooden cutting board. Place ½ tablespoon of the mint and ½ tablespoon of the cilantro along the bottom third of the wrapper. Top with one-eighth of the noodles, avocado, spinach, bell pepper, carrot, and chicken. Fold the bottom of the rice paper up and over the filling. Fold in the sides and continue rolling until the roll is sealed completely. Repeat with the remaining wrappers and fillings. Cut each roll in half crosswise and serve 2 rolls per person, with the sauce.

WALNUT-CRUSTED CHICKEN BREASTS WITH POMEGRANATE SYRUP

No wonder pomegranates are popular: They're a great source of antioxidants, and they taste wonderful, like a combination of apples, mixed berries, and citrus—a fruit salad in a glass! With so many pomegranate juice blends now available, feel free to experiment with your favorite in this recipe; just make sure to use a brand that's labeled 100 percent fruit juice.

MAKES 4 SERVINGS

1 egg

1 tablespoon water

½ cup walnuts, finely chopped

¼ cup whole grain gluten-free bread crumbs

½ teaspoon unrefined sea salt

4 boneless, skinless organic chicken breast halves (5 ounces each)

2 cups pomegranate juice

1 tablespoon honey

2 teaspoons minced crystallized ginger

6 cups mesclun or mixed greens

Preheat the oven to 425°F. Coat a baking sheet with cooking spray. In a shallow dish, whisk the egg with the water. In another shallow dish, combine the walnuts, bread crumbs, and salt. Dip the chicken into the egg mixture and then into the nut mixture. Place on the baking sheet. Bake, turning once, for 15 minutes, or until a thermometer inserted in the thickest portion registers 165°F and the juices run clear. Let rest for 10 minutes, then slice the breasts.

Meanwhile, in a small pan over medium-high heat, combine the pomegranate juice, honey, and ginger and boil for 15 minutes, or until reduced by half. Remove from the heat and set aside. Arrange the greens on 4 plates. Place the chicken on top and drizzle with the pomegranate syrup.

SPICE-RUBBED CHICKEN WITH MILLET PILAF

This easy one-dish meal features millet, a gluten-free grain that provides 2 grams of fiber per 1-cup serving. If you enjoy nutty flavors in your meals, try toasting the millet in a dry skillet until lightly browned before using it in this recipe.

MAKES 4 SERVINGS

1 teaspoon ground paprika

1 teaspoon ground cumin

¾ teaspoon unrefined sea salt

4 bone-in, skinless organic chicken thighs (about 1½ pounds)

2 tablespoons olive oil, divided

1 onion, chopped

2 cloves garlic, minced

1 cup millet

1 can (14.5 ounces) diced tomatoes, drained

1 cup reduced-sodium organic chicken broth

1 bay leaf

¼ teaspoon freshly ground black pepper

1 cup frozen peas, thawed

In a small bowl, combine the paprika, cumin, and salt. Rub on all surfaces of the chicken thighs. In a Dutch oven or large saucepan over medium-high heat, heat 1 tablespoon of the oil. Cook the chicken for 6 minutes, turning once, or until browned. Remove to a plate.

Add the remaining 1 tablespoon oil to the same pan and reduce the heat to medium. Cook the onion and garlic, stirring, for 3 minutes. Stir in the millet, tomatoes, broth, and bay leaf. Nestle the chicken into the mixture and sprinkle with the pepper. Increase the heat to medium high and bring to a boil. Reduce the heat to low, cover, and simmer for 20 minutes, or until the millet is tender and a thermometer inserted in the thickest portion of the chicken registers 170°F and the juices run clear. Remove from the heat and stir in the peas. Cover and let stand for 10 minutes. Discard the bay leaf.

SMOKY GRILLED CHICKEN WITH TOMATO CHUTNEY

Sweet and zesty, this chutney is delicious over chicken breasts. Try it on tacos, too. If you like, make it ahead and refrigerate for up to 1 week. The flavors will only improve.

MAKES 4 SERVINGS

CHICKEN

2 cloves garlic, minced

Grated peel and juice of 1 lime

2 teaspoons olive oil

1 teaspoon dried oregano

1 teaspoon ground cumin

¾ teaspoon unrefined sea salt

½ teaspoon freshly ground black pepper

4 boneless, skinless organic chicken breast halves

CHUTNEY

2 teaspoons olive oil

1 red onion, finely chopped

1 bell pepper, finely chopped

1 canned chipotle chile pepper in adobo sauce, seeded and minced

1 can (14.5 ounces) diced tomatoes, drained

½ cup pomegranate juice

1 tablespoon honey

½ cup golden raisins

¼ cup dried cranberries

½ teaspoon unrefined sea salt

¼ cup slivered almonds

To make the chicken: In a large resealable plastic bag, combine the garlic, lime peel and juice, oil, oregano, cumin, salt, and black pepper. Add the chicken and seal. Refrigerate for up to 2 hours, turning occasionally.

Preheat the grill. Remove the chicken from the marinade. Discard the marinade. Grill the chicken for 10 to 12 minutes, turning once, or until a thermometer inserted in the thickest portion registers 165°F and the juices run clear.

To make the chutney: In a medium saucepan over medium-high heat, heat the oil. Cook the onion and bell pepper, stirring, for 5 minutes, or until the onion is tender. Add the chipotle pepper, tomatoes, pomegranate juice, honey, raisins, cranberries, and salt. Reduce the heat to low, cover, and simmer for 10 minutes. Remove from the heat and stir in the almonds. The chutney can be made up to 24 hours ahead of time. Bring to room temperature before serving with the chicken.

Desserts

STRAWBERRY-BLUEBERRY PUDDING

This is a quick and easy way to satisfy a sweet tooth. From fridge to fantastic in under 5 minutes!

MAKES 2 SERVINGS

1 avocado, peeled and pitted

Juice of ½ lemon

½ cup frozen blueberries

½ cup fresh strawberries, hulled

In a food processor, place the avocado, lemon juice, blueberries, and strawberries. Process until smooth. (Alternatively, use a hand blender.) Serve immediately.

DAIRY-FREE VANILLA ICE CREAM

This is the fastest, easiest, and most nutritious ice cream you can make. And it tastes great. If you don't have an ice cream maker, you can freeze it in ice pop molds to make delicious vanilla ice cream pops.

MAKES 2 TO 4 SERVINGS

⅔ cup unsalted raw cashews

4 fresh Medjool dates, pitted (or more if you prefer a sweeter ice cream)

2½ cups unsweetened almond milk

2 teaspoons pure vanilla extract or vanilla powder (see note)

In a blender, place the cashews, dates, almond milk, and vanilla extract or powder. Blend until smooth. Pour into an ice cream maker and follow the manufacturer's instructions. Serve immediately.

Note: Vanilla powder is ground vanilla beans and is not the same as vanilla sugar.

CHOCOLATE TRUFFLES

Forget the double boilers, thermometer, and delicate techniques required to make traditional truffles. These delectable bites take minimal effort and can be made in less than 15 minutes. They satisfy even the worst chocolate cravings, yet are packed with calcium, magnesium, and even fiber!

MAKES 12

⅔ cup raw almonds

6 fresh Medjool dates, pitted

2 tablespoons unsweetened cocoa powder + additional to coat the truffles

In a food processor, finely grind the almonds. Add the dates and 2 tablespoons of cocoa and process until smooth.

Take a large teaspoonful of the almond-chocolate mixture and roll it into a ball between your palms. Roll the ball in additional cocoa to coat.

Continue until all of the almond-chocolate mixture is used.

PLUM PUDDING

The key to the creamy texture and sweet taste of this pudding is using fruit that is really ripe. I like using black plums, since they are so sweet. Papayas are ripe when their skin turns quite yellow and the flesh yields slightly to the touch. These fruits offer an outstanding combination of delicious taste and excellent nutrition.

MAKES 2 TO 4 SERVINGS

4 ripe plums, skin left on, pitted

½ small papaya, peeled and seeded, or about 1 cup cubed papaya

1 teaspoon unpasteurized honey

In a blender, combine the plums, papaya, and honey. Blend until smooth. Chill before serving.

PEACH-PINEAPPLE ICE CREAM

This is one of the most delicious ice creams I've ever tasted. It's so good, no one will know it's healthy. Yet it couldn't be easier to make. It takes about 5 minutes plus a couple of hours of freezing time (less if you're using an ice cream maker).

MAKES 2 TO 4 SERVINGS

2 cups cubed pineapple

2 peaches, skin left on, pitted and sliced

1 teaspoon unpasteurized honey

In a blender, combine the pineapple, peaches, and honey. Blend until smooth. Pour into empty ice cube trays and place in the freezer for 2 to 3 hours.

Serve as is or whip in a food processor just prior to serving.

STRAWBERRY GELATO

This delicious treat has a way of disappearing in a hurry. Once you've tasted it, you'll completely understand how it makes its disappearing act. In addition to being packed with brain-building nutrients, it's a cinch to make, so you can have this delicious soft-serve gelato ready to enjoy in only a few minutes.

MAKES 4 SERVINGS

1½ cups cubed fresh pineapple

2 cups frozen strawberries

1 cup frozen cranberries

1 cup water

In a blender, combine the pineapple, strawberries, cranberries, and water. Blend until smooth. (If your blender has a plunger attachment, you can use it to coax the ingredients to blend together smoothly.) Serve immediately.

APPLE AND ALMOND MEDLEY

Topped with just a light, crunchy coating of almonds, these sweet and spicy apples are the perfect way to end a special meal. And since eating an apple a day has so many health benefits, what have you got to lose? An apple sure is more delicious than a pill.

MAKES 4 SERVINGS

2 tablespoons sliced almonds

4 Granny Smith apples

2 tablespoons lemon juice

1 teaspoon olive oil

¼ cup apple cider

1 tablespoon maple syrup

¼ teaspoon grated lemon peel

¼ teaspoon vanilla extract

¼ teaspoon ground cinnamon

¼ teaspoon ground cloves

In a dry skillet over medium heat, toast the almonds, shaking often, for 3 to 5 minutes, or until fragrant and golden. Set aside. Peel, core, and slice the apples. In a large bowl, toss the apples with the lemon juice. In a large skillet over medium-high heat, heat the oil. Cook the apples, stirring, for 2 minutes. Reduce the heat to low, cover, and simmer, stirring occasionally, for 5 to 8 minutes, or until the apples are just tender. Using a slotted spoon, carefully divide among 4 dessert dishes. To the skillet, add the cider, maple syrup, lemon peel, vanilla, cinnamon, and cloves. Increase the heat to medium high and cook, stirring constantly, until syrupy. Spoon over the apples. Sprinkle with the reserved almonds.

STRAWBERRY-CHOCOLATE ROYALE

This sinfully delicious dessert is perfect for a romantic evening or to satisfy a chocolate craving. It can be whipped up in a matter of minutes.

MAKES 2 SERVINGS

1 large avocado, pitted and halved

3 tablespoons organic unsweetened cocoa powder

1 tablespoon pure maple syrup

1 banana, sliced

6–10 strawberries, hulled and sliced

Scoop the avocado flesh into a medium bowl.

Add the cocoa powder and maple syrup. Using a hand blender, mash the avocado, cocoa, and maple syrup together until the cocoa powder is integrated. Blend until smooth.

To serve, place a scoop of the chocolate-avocado mixture into the bottoms of 2 wine glasses. Add a layer of banana slices, then a layer of strawberry slices. Continue layering the chocolate mixture with the bananas and strawberries until all ingredients are used.

Tip: This dessert is best when served immediately.

60 Seconds to Boost Your Brain Power
1-Week Meal Plan

Day 1

BREAKFAST

Blueberry Pancakes (page 210) and Water-Berry Juice (page 226)

MIDMORNING SNACK

Hummus (page 233) and vegetable crudités

LUNCH

Veggie and Wild Rice Soup (page 234) and Southwestern Bruschetta (page 228)

MIDAFTERNOON SNACK

Apple and a handful of raw, unsalted almonds

DINNER

Lentil Burgers (page 263) and Citrus-Ginger Salad (page 250)

DESSERT (OPTIONAL)

Chocolate Truffles (page 293)

Day 2

BREAKFAST

Gluten-Free Toast with Coco-Almond Butter and Peaches (page 217)

MIDMORNING SNACK

Celery sticks with almond butter

LUNCH

Thai Noodle Salad (page 252)

MIDAFTERNOON SNACK

Peach, plum, or apricot

DINNER

Grilled Salmon with Plum-Blueberry-Grape Salsa (page 279)

Day 3

BREAKFAST

Brain-Building Eggless Scramble (page 211)

MIDMORNING SNACK

½ cup fresh or frozen blueberries or 10 cherries

LUNCH

Dairy-Free Pasta Alfredo with Asparagus (page 274) and a green salad

MIDAFTERNOON SNACK

Pinto bean chips (available in most health food stores) with
Avo-Salsa (page 231)

DINNER

Warm Black Bean Salad (page 246) and Roasted Carrot Soup (page 236)

DESSERT (OPTIONAL)

Dairy-Free Vanilla Ice Cream (page 292)

Day 4

BREAKFAST

Apple-Cinnamon-Walnut Oats (page 216) and Almond Milk (page 223)

MIDMORNING SNACK

Raw almonds and/or fresh, frozen, or freeze-dried blueberries

LUNCH

Southwestern Bruschetta (page 228) and Warm Black Bean Salad (page 246)

MIDAFTERNOON SNACK

Bunch of purple grapes or a pomegranate

DINNER

Pineapple-Basil Rice (page 269) and Roasted Carrot Soup (page 236) and Green Goddess Juice (page 227)

DESSERT (OPTIONAL)

Strawberry Gelato (page 296)

Day 5

BREAKFAST

Superbrainiac Breakfast Smoothie (page 212) and Gluten-Free Toast (page 217) with Coco-Almond Butter (page 218)

MIDMORNING SNACK

Iced Pomegranate Green Tea (page 221) and a handful of raw, unsalted walnuts

LUNCH

Salade de Provence (page 247) with cooked chicken breast

MIDAFTERNOON SNACK

Pineapple-Basil Rice (page 269) or Super-Health-Boosting Pumpkin Spice "Latte" (page 224)

DINNER

Basil-Lettuce-Tomato-Pepper (BLTP) Sandwiches (page 264) with a green salad

DESSERT (OPTIONAL)

Strawberry-Chocolate Royale (page 298)

Day 6

BREAKFAST

Blueberry Pancakes (page 210)

MIDMORNING SNACK

Super-Health-Boosting Pumpkin Spice "Latte" (page 224)

LUNCH

Green Bean Ragout (page 275) and Lentil Burgers (page 263)

MIDAFTERNOON SNACK

Ginger Lemonade (page 220) and Hummus with crudités (page 233)

DINNER

Thai Noodle Salad (page 252) and Green Goddess Juice (page 227)

DESSERT (OPTIONAL)

Peach-Pineapple Ice Cream (page 295)

Day 7

BREAKFAST

Brain-Building Eggless Scramble (page 211) and Almond Milk (page 223)

MIDMORNING SNACK

Iced Pomegranate Green Tea (page 221) and a handful of raw, unsalted almonds

LUNCH

Quick Spelt Bread (page 219) or your favorite gluten-free bread with Citrus-Ginger Salad (page 250)

MIDAFTERNOON SNACK

Black bean chips and Brain-Building Salsa (page 231)

DINNER

Grilled Salmon with Plum-Blueberry-Grape Salsa (page 279)

DESSERT (OPTIONAL)

Strawberry-Blueberry Pudding (page 291)

ENDNOTES

Chapter 1

1   Mayo Clinic Staff, "Diseases and Conditions: Traumatic Brain Injury," May 15, 2014, mayoclinic.org/diseases-conditions/traumatic-brain-injury/basics/symptoms /con-20029302.

2   Joseph Mercola, "Monsanto's Roundup Herbicide May Be Most Important Factor in Development of Autism and Other Chronic Disease," June 9, 2013, articles.mercola. com/sites/articles/archive/2013/06/09/monsanto-roundup-herbicide.aspx.

3   H. Chen, "Anti-Inflammatory Drugs Dramatically Reduce Parkinson's Risk," *Archives of Neurology* 60 (2003): 1059–64.

4   J. J. Gagne and M. C. Power, "Anti-Inflammatory Drugs and Risk of Parkinson's Disease," *Neurology* 74, no. 10 (March 2010): 995–1002, ncbi.nlm.nih.gov/pmc /articles/PMC2848103/.

5   Kate Lowenstein, "Is Inflammation What's Causing Your Depression?" March 23, 2014, prevention.com/health/health-concerns/link-between-inflammation-pain-and-depression.

6   Ibid.

Chapter 2

1   Nancy Appleton, PhD, *Lick the Sugar Habit* (New York: Avery, 1988).

2   W. Jiang et al., "Dairy Food Intake and Risk of Parkinson's Disease: A Dose-Response Meta-Analysis of Prospective Cohort Studies," *European Journal of Epidemiology* 29, no. 9 (September 2014): 613–19, ncbi.nlm.nih.gov/pubmed/24894826.

3   R. Panusch et al., "Food Induced (Allergic) Arthritis: Inflammatory Arthritis Exacerbated by Milk," *Arthritis and Rheumatism* 29, no. 2 (February 1986): 220–26, onlinelibrary.wiley.com/doi/10.1002/art.1780290210/abstract.

4   M. Heid, "Study: Common Anxiety, Sleeping Meds Linked to Alzheimer's," September 9, 2014, prevention.com/health/health-concerns/common-medications-linked-alzheimers?cid=socPVNN_20140910_31335366.

5   S. Eckelkamp, "7 Ways to Prevent Alzheimer's Disease," August 28, 2013, abcnews.go.com /Health/Wellness/ways-prevent-alzheimers-disease/story?id=20086157.

6   J. Robert Hatherill, PhD, *The Brain Gate* (Washington, DC: Lifeline Press, 2003), 81–82.

7   Joseph Mercola, DO, "Avoiding Artificial Sweeteners? This Study Will Surprise You," September 20, 2011, articles.mercola.com/sites/articles/archive/2011/09/20/why-are-millions-of-americans-getting-this-synthetic-sweetener-in-their-drinking-water.aspx?e_cid=20110920_DNL_art_1.

8   Randall Fitzgerald, *The Hundred-Year Lie* (New York: Plume, 2007).

9   Betty Kovacs, "Artificial Sweeteners: Health and Disease Prevention," medicinenet.com/artificial_sweeteners/article.htm.

10 Joseph Mercola, DO, "Could Deficiency in B Vitamins Be the Key Factor Spiking the Rise of Dementia and Alzheimer's?" September 28, 2010, articles.mercola.com/sites/articles/archive/2010/09/28/high-doses-of-b-vitamins-can-reduce-brain-shrinkage-memory-loss.aspx.

Chapter 3

1   S. Dunlevy, "High Sugar Diet Can Damage Your Brain in a Week, University of NSW Survey," December 17, 2013, news.com.au/lifestyle/food/high-sugar-diet-can-damage-your-brain-in-a-week-university-of-nsw-survey/story-fneuz8wn-1226784379678.

2   D. DiSalvo, "What Eating Too Much Sugar Does to Your Brain," *Psychology Today*, April 27, 2012, psychologytoday.com/blog/neuronarrative/201204/what-eating-too-much-sugar-does-your-brain.

3   Ibid.

4   R. Fitzgerald, *The Hundred-Year Lie: How to Protect Yourself from the Chemicals That Are Destroying Your Health* (New York: Penguin, 2006), 72.

5   Ibid., 107.

6   R. Seroka and A. Babb, "Hold the Diet Soda? Sweetened Drinks Linked to Depression," American Academy of Neurology 65th Annual Meeting Abstract, January 8, 2013, aan.com/PressRoom/home/GetDigitalAsset/10430.

7   K. Rycerz and J. E. Jaworska-Adamu, "Effects of Aspartame Metabolites on Astrocytes and Neurons," *Folia Neuropathologica* 51, no. 1 (2013): 10–17, ncbi.nlm.nih.gov/pubmed/23553132.

8   C. Nordqvist, "What Is Serotonin? What Does Serotonin Do?" February 12, 2015, medicalnewstoday.com/articles/232248.php.

9   "What Is Serotonin and What Does It Do?" macalester.edu/academics/psychology/whathap/ubnrp/placebo/serotonin2.html.

10 Mandy Oaklander, "7 Side Effects of Drinking Diet Soda," August 21, 2012, prevention.com/food/healthy-eating-tips/diet-soda-bad-you?slide=1.

11 Ibid.

12 Ibid.

13 Ibid.

14 Ibid.

15 Ibid.

16 "Epilepsy Drug Helps Fight Parkinson's," *Neurology* (April 24, 2000).

17 P. Fitzgerald, *The Detox Solution: The Missing Link to Radiant Health, Abundant Energy, Ideal Weight, and Peace of Mind* (Santa Monica, CA: Illumination Press, 2001), 73.

18 R. L. Blaylock, MD, *Excitotoxins: The Taste That Kills* (Santa Fe, NM: Health Press, 1997), 116.

19 Ibid.

20 J. Barbaresko et al., "Dietary Pattern Analysis and Biomarkers of Low-Grade Inflammation: A Systematic Literature Review," *Nutrition Reviews* 71, no. 8 (August 2013): 511–27, onlinelibrary.wiley.com/doi/10.1111/nure.12035/abstract.

21 E. Angvall, "Are Heavy Metals Evildoers in Alzheimer's Disease?" *AARP: The Magazine*, August 23, 2013, blog.aarp.org/2013/08/23/are-heavy-metals-evildoers-in -alzheimers-disease/.

22 J. Robert Hatherill, PhD, *The Brain Gate* (Washington, DC: Lifeline Press, 2003), 133.

23 Ibid., 149.

24 D. Perlmutter, MD, FANC, and Carol Colman, *The Better Brain Book* (New York: Riverhead Books, 2004), 150.

25 J. Robert Hatherill, PhD, *The Brain Gate* (Washington, DC: Lifeline Press, 2003), 129.

26 W. H. Philpott, MD, and Dwight K. Kalita, PhD, *Brain Allergies: The Psychonutrient and Magnetic Connections* (Los Angeles: Keats Publishing, 2000), 68–69.

27 D. Perlmutter, MD, FANC, and Carol Colman, *The Better Brain Book* (New York: Riverhead Books, 2004), 150.

28 David Suzuki Foundation, "'Dirty Dozen' Cosmetic Chemicals to Avoid," davidsuzuki.org/issues/health/science/toxics/dirty-dozen-cosmetic-chemicals /?gclid=CKPI2rPgvsECFQcSMwodfG4A3Q.

29 Ibid.

30 David Suzuki Foundation, "DEA," davidsuzuki.org/issues/health/science/toxics /chemicals-in-your-cosmetics---dea/.

31 Breast Cancer Fund, "Pthalates," breastcancerfund.org/clear-science/radiation -chemicals-and-breast-cancer/phthalates.html.

32 David Suzuki Foundation, "'Dirty Dozen' Cosmetic Chemicals to Avoid," davidsuzuki.org/issues/health/science/toxics/dirty-dozen-cosmetic-chemicals/ ?gclid=CKPI2rPgvsECFQcSMwodfG4A3Q.

33 David Suzuki Foundation, "Parabens," davidsuzuki.org/issues/health/science/toxics/ chemicals-in-your-cosmetics---parabens/.

34 David Suzuki Foundation, "'Dirty Dozen' Cosmetic Chemicals to Avoid," davidsuzuki.org/issues/health/science/toxics/dirty-dozen-cosmetic-chemicals/?gclid =CKPI2rPgvsECFQcSMwodfG4A3Q.

35 "Cancer-Causing Toxic Chemical Ingredients in Cosmetics and Skin Care Products," health-report.co.uk/ingredients-directory.htm#Stearalkonium%20Chloride.

36 Ibid.

37 "Material Safety Data Sheet: Benzyl Acetate MSDS," May 21, 2013, sciencelab.com /msds.php?msdsId=9923066.

38 A. Cohen, S. Janssen, and G. Solomon, "Clearing the Air: Hidden Hazards of Air Fresheners," September 2001, nrdc.org/health/home/airfresheners/airfresheners.pdf.

39 S. Neese, "Common Plasticizer Alters an Important Memory System in Male Rat Brains," September 2, 2011, environmentalhealthnews.org/ehs/newscience/2011/08 /2011-0901-phthalate-rats-hipocampus/.

40 "Chemical Effects on the Brain and Behaviour," chemicalwatch.com/11011/chemical-effects-on-the-brain-and-behaviour.

41 "Air 'Fresheners'," silentmenace.com/-Air_Fresheners.html.

42 Ibid.

Chapter 4

1 S. Subash et al., "Pomegranate from Oman Eliminates the Brain Oxidative Damage in Transgenic Mouse Model Alzheimer's Disease," *Journal of Traditional and Complementary Medicine* 4, no. 4 (October 2014): 232–38, ncbi.nlm.nih.gov/pubmed/25379464.

2 A. A. Ahmed et al., "Pomegranate Extract Modulates Processing of Amyloid B Precursor Protein in an Aged Alzheimer's Disease Animal Model," *Current Alzheimer's Research* 11, no. 9 (October 1, 2014): 834–43, ncbi.nlm.nih.gov/pubmed/25274111.

3 M. A. Ahmed et al., "Pomegranate Extract Protects against Cerebral Ischemia/ Reperfusion Injury and Preserves Brain DNA Integrity in Rats," *Life Sciences* 110, no. 2 (August 21, 2014): 61–69, ncbi.nlm.nih.gov/pubmed/25010842.

4 M. Rosenblat et al., "Pomegranate Phytosterol (B-sitosterol) and Polyphenolic Antioxidant (Punicalagin) Addition to Statin, Significantly Protected against

Macrophage Foam Cells Formation," *Atherosclerosis* 226, no. 1 (January 2013): 110–17, ncbi.nlm.nih.gov/pubmed/23141585.

5   A. S. Matthew et al., "Acute Effects of Pomegranate Extract on Postprandial Lipaemia, Vascular Function, and Blood Pressure," *Plant Foods for Human Nutrition* 67, no. 4 (December 2012): 351–57, ncbi.nlm.nih.gov/pubmed/23093401.

6   V. Tapias et al., "Pomegranate Juice Exacerbates Oxidative Stress and Nigrostriatal Degeneration in Parkinson's Disease," *Neurobiology of Aging* 35, no. 5 (May 2014): 1162–76, ncbi.nlm.nih.gov/pubmed/24315037.

7   M. Cekmen et al., "Pomegranate Extract Attenuates Gentamicin-Induced Nephrotoxicity in Rats by Reducing Oxidative Stress," *Renal Failure* 35, no. 2 (2013): 268–74, ncbi.nlm.nih.gov/pubmed/23176634.

8   M. Pirinççioglu et al., "The Protective Role of Pomegranate Juice against Carbon Tetrachloride-Induced Oxidative Stress in Rats," *Toxicology and Industrial Health* 30, no. 10 (November 2014): 910–18, ncbi.nlm.nih.gov/pubmed/23160382.

9   S. Medjacovic and A. Jungbauer, "Pomegranate: A Fruit That Ameliorates Metabolic Syndrome," *Food and Function* 4, no. 1 (January 2013): 19–39, ncbi.nlm.nih.gov /pubmed/23060097.

10 D. Dey et al., "Pomegranate Pericarp Extract Enhances the Antibacterial Activity of Ciprofloxacin against Extended Spectrum B-Lactamase (ESBL) and Mettalo-B-Lactamase (MBL) Producing Gram-Negative Bacilli," *Food and Chemical Toxicology* 50, no. 12 (December 2012): 4302–9, ncbi.nlm.nih.gov/pubmed/22982804.

11 L. Wang et al., "Specific Pomegranate Juice Components As Potential Inhibitors of Prostate Cancer Metastasis," *Translational Oncology* 5, no. 5 (October 2012): 344–55, ncbi.nlm.nih.gov/pubmed/23066443.

12 A. Rocha et al., "Pomegranate Juice and Specific Components Inhibit Cell and Molecular Processes Critical for Metastasis of Breast Cancer," *Breast Cancer Research and Treatment* 136, no. 3 (December 2012): 647–58, ncbi.nlm.nih.gov/pubmed /23065001.

13 E. Devries et al., "Known and Potential New Risk Factors for Skin Cancer in European Population: A Multi-Centre Case-Control Study," *British Journal of Dermatology* 167, sup. 2 (August 2012): 1–13, ncbi.nlm.nih.gov/pubmed/22881582.

14 Z. Li and P. Srivastava, "Heat Shock Proteins," *Current Protocols in Immunology* (2004), ncbi.nlm.nih.gov/pubmed/18432918.

15 Rachael Moeller Gorman, "Food for Thought: Can Healthy Eating Help Your Brain Stay Sharp?" *Eating Well* (April/May 2006).

16 Michael Colgan, PhD, "Save Your Brain," *Vista*.

17 "Curry Ingredient May Stop Alzheimer's." *Medical News Today* (September 9, 2004), medicalnewstoday.com/medicalnews.php?newsid=13116.

18 P. Wang et al., "Mechanisms and Effects of Curcumin on Spatial Learning and Memory Improvement in APPswe/PS1dE9 Mice," *Journal of Neuroscience Research* 92, no. 2 (February 2014): 218–31, ncbi.nlm.nih.gov/pubmed/24273069.

19 N. Hishikawa et al., "Effect of Turmeric on Alzheimer's Disease with Behavioral and Psychological Symptoms of Dementia," *Ayu* 33, no. 4 (October 2012): 499–504, ncbi.nlm.nih.gov/pubmed/23723666.

20 Michelle Schoffro Cook, *Healing Injuries the Natural Way: How to Mend Bones, Muscles, Tendons, and More* (Toronto: Your Health Press, 2004).

21 Rachael Moeller Gorman, "Food for Thought: Can Healthy Eating Help Your Brain Stay Sharp?" *Eating Well*, April/May 2006.

22 H. Checkoway et al., "Parkinson's Disease Risks Associated with Cigarette Smoking, Alcohol Consumption, and Caffeine Intake," *American Journal of Epidemiology* 155, no. 8 (2002): 732–38.

23 J. Robert Hatherhill, *The Brain Gate* (Washington, DC: LifeLine Press, 2003), 88.

24 H. S. Kim et al., "Epigallocatechin Gallate (EGCG) Stimulates Autophagy in Vascular Epithelial Cells: A Potential Role for Reducing Lipid Accumulation," *Journal of Biological Chemistry* 288, no. 31 (August 2, 2013): 22693–705, ncbi.nlm.nih.gov /pubmed/23754277.

25 G. Webster Ross et al., "Association of Coffee and Caffeine Intake with the Risk of Parkinson Disease," *Journal of the American Medical Association* 283, no. 20 (May 24/31, 2000): 2674–79.

26 J. Robert Hatherhill, *The Brain Gate* (Washington, DC: LifeLine Press, 2003), 150.

27 George Mateljan, "The World's Healthiest Foods: Kidney Beans," whfoods.com /genpage.php?tname=foodspice&dbid=87.

28 Rachael Moeller Gorman, "Food for Thought: Can Healthy Eating Help Your Brain Stay Sharp?" *Eating Well* (April/May 2006).

29 R. Remington et al., "Apple Juice Improved Behavioral but Not Cognitive Symptoms in Moderate-to-Late Stage Alzheimer's Disease in an Open-Label Pilot Study," *American Journal of Alzheimer's Disease and Other Dementias* 25, no. 4 (June 2010): 367–71, ncbi.nlm.nih.gov/pubmed/20338990.

30 F. Tchantchou et al., "Dietary Supplementation with Apple Juice Concentrate Alleviates the Compensatory Increase in Glutathione Synthase Transcription and Activity that Accompanies Dietary- and Genetically-Induced Oxidative Stress," *Journal*

of Nutrition, Health & Aging 8, no. 6 (2004): 492–96, ncbi.nlm.nih.gov/pubmed /15543422.

31 A. Chan et al., "Apple Juice Concentrate Maintains Acetylcholine Levels Following Dietary Compromise," *Journal of Alzheimer's Disease* 9, no. 3 (August 2006): 287–91, ncbi.nlm.nih.gov/pubmed/16914839.

32 Kendra Cherry, "What is Acetylcholine?" psychology.about.com/od/aindex/g /acetylcholine.htm.

33 A. D. M. Briggs, "A Statin a Day Keeps the Doctor Away: Comparative Proverb Assessment Modelling Study" *British Medical Journal* 343 (December 17, 2013): f7267, bmj.com/content/347/bmj.f7267.

34 M. Naziroglu et al., "Apple Cider Vinegar Modulates Serum Lipid Profile, Erythrocyte, Kidney, and Liver Membrane Oxidative Stress in Ovariectomized Mice Fed High Cholesterol," *Journal of Membrane Biology* 247, no. 8 (August 2014): 667–73, ncbi.nlm.nih.gov/pubmed/24894721.

35 J. A. Laranjinha et al., "Reactivity of Dietary Phenolic Acids with Peroxyl Radicals: Antioxidant Activity upon Low Density Lipoprotein Peroxidation," *Biochemical Pharmacology* 48, no. 3 (August 3, 1994): 487–94, ncbi.nlm.nih.gov/pubmed/8068036.

36 E. Ostman et al., "Vinegar Supplementation Lowers Glucose and Insulin Responses and Increases Satiety after a Bread Meal in Healthy Subjects," *European Journal of Clinical Nutrition* 59, no. 9 (September 2005): 983–88, ncbi.nlm.nih.gov/pubmed /16015276.

37 T. Kondo et al., "Vinegar Intake Reduces Body Weight, Body Fat Mass, and Serum Triglycerides in Obese Japanese Subjects," *Bioscience, Biotechnology, and Biochemistry* 73, no. 8 (August 2009): 1837–43, ncbi.nlm.nih.gov/pubmed/19661687.

38 H. Chen et al., "Nonsteroidal Anti-Inflammatory Drugs and the Risk of Parkinson Disease," *Archive of Neurology* 60, no. 8 (2003): 1059–64.

39 Michelle Schoffro Cook, DNM, DAc, CNC, *Healing Injuries the Natural Way* (Toronto: Your Health Press, Inc., 2004), 29.

40 Bharat B. Aggarwal, PhD with Debora Yost, *Healing Spices* (New York: Sterling Publishing, 2011), 138.

41 S. M. Poulose et al., "Role of Walnuts in Maintaining Brain Health with Age," *Journal of Nutrition* 144, sup. 4 (April 2014): 561S–66S, ncbi.nlm.nih.gov/pubmed/24500933.

42 Julia Westbrook, "Walnuts Show Promise for Alzheimer's Prevention," *Prevention*, October 27, 2014, rodalenews.com/walnuts-alzheimers.

43 J. Robert Hatherhill, *The Brain Gate* (Washington, DC: LifeLine Press, 2003), 88–89.

44 George Mateljan, "The World's Healthiest Foods: Rosemary," whfoods.com/genpage. php?tname=foodspice&dbid=75.

45 M. Ozarowski et al., "Rosmarinus Officinalis L. Leaf Extract Improves Memory Impairment and Affects Acetylcholinesterase and Butyrylcholinesterase Activities in Rat Brain," ncbi.nlm.nih.gov/pubmed/24080468.

46 Gyeong Chae et al., "Effect of Rosmarinus Officinalis L. on MMP-9, MCP-1 Levels, and Cell Migration in RAW 267.4 and Smooth Muscle Cells," *Journal of Medicinal Food* 15, no. 10 (October 2012): 879–86, ncbi.nlm.nih.gov/pmc/articles/PMC3466913/.

47 K. Murata et al. "Promotion of Hair Growth by Rosmarinus officinalis Leaf Extract," *Phytotherapy Research* 27, no. 2 (February 2013): 212–17, ncbi.nlm.nih.gov/pubmed /22517595.

48 S. M. Petiwala et al., "Rosemary (Rosmarinus officinalis) Extract Modulates CHOP/ GADD153 to Promote Androgen Receptor Degradation and Decreases Xenograft Tumor Growth," *PLoS One* 9, no. 3 (March 2014): e89772, ncbi.nlm.nih.gov/pubmed /24598693.

49 "Tomatoes and Stroke Prevention: New Evidence Shows Lycopene Is Not Just a Cancer Fighter," *Harvard Health Letter* 38, no. 4 (February 2013): 4, ncbi.nlm.nih.gov/pubmed /23841168.

50 "Red Wine Molecule May Protect Brain from Alzheimer's," *Reuters Health* (December 31, 2003).

51 Joseph Mercola, DO, "Resveratrol Boosts Brain Flow," May 27, 2010, articles.mercola .com/sites/articles/archive/2010/05/27/resveratrol-boosts-brain-blood-flow.aspx.

52 "Resveratrol," phytochemicals.info/phytochemicals/resveratrol.php.

53 M. Soman, "10 Surprising Health Facts about Caffeine," *Good Housekeeping*, goodhousekeeping.com/health/womens-health/caffeine.

54 J. L. Cechella et al., "Moderate Swimming Exercise and Caffeine Supplementation Reduced the Levels of Inflammatory Cytokines without Causing Oxidative Stress in Tissues of Middle-Aged Rats," *Amino Acids* 46, no. 5 (May 2014): 1187–95, ncbi.nlm.nih.gov/pubmed/24481487.

55 M. Soman, "10 Surprising Health Facts about Caffeine," *Good Housekeeping*, goodhousekeeping.com/health/womens-health/caffeine.

56 H. Kou et al., "Maternal Glucocorticoid Elevation and Associated Blood Metabonome Changes Might Be Involved in Metabolic Programming of Intrauterine Growth Retardation in Rats Exposed to Caffeine Prenatally," *Toxicology and Applied Pharmacology* 275, no. 2 (March 2014): 79–87, ncbi.nlm.nih.gov /pubmed/24463096.

57 Ibid.

58 K. Ritchie et al., "The Association between Caffeine and Cognitive Decline: Examining Alternative Causal Hypotheses," *International Psychogeriatrics*, 26, no. 4 (April 2014): 581–90, ncbi.nlm.nih.gov/pubmed/24423697.

59 M. Oatman, "9 Things You Should Know about Your Caffeine Habit," *Mother Jones*, March 5, 2014, motherjones.com/environment/2014/03/caffeine-murray-carpenter -energy-drink-keurig-cup-coffee.

60 "Coffee," Verité, verite.org/Commodities/Coffee.

61 M. Greger, "Is Potassium Sorbate Bad for You?" October 18, 2011, nutritionfacts.org /video/is-potassium-sorbate-bad-for-you/.

62 M. Soman, "10 Surprising Health Facts about Caffeine," *Good Housekeeping*, goodhousekeeping.com/health/womens-health/caffeine.

63 Ibid.

64 G. Mateljan, "What's New and Beneficial about Onions," The World's Healthiest Foods, whfoods.com/genpage.php?tname=foodspice&dbid=45.

65 Michael Castleman, *The New Healing Herbs* (New York: Bantam Books, 2002), 286.

66 Neelima B. Chauhan, "Effect of Aged Garlic Extract on APP Processing and Tau Phosphyloration in Alzheimer's Transgenic Model Tg2576," *Journal of Ethnopharmacology* 108, no. 3 (December 6, 2006): 385–94, sciencedirect.com /science/article/pii/S0378874106002911.

67 Neelima B. Chauhan and J. Sandoval, "Amelioration of Early Cognitive Deficits by Aged Garlic Extract in Alzheimer's Transgenic Mice," *Phytotherapy Research* 21, no. 7 (July 2007): 629–40, ncbi.nlm.nih.gov/pubmed/17380553.

Chapter 5

1 "Sleep Makes Your Memories Stronger," Association for Psychological Science (November 12, 2010), psychologicalscience.org/index.php/news/releases/sleep-makes -your-memories-stronger.html.

2 "Live Well, Resist Alzheimer's," *Medical News Today*, July 20, 2004, medicalnewstoday .com/medicalnews.php?newsid=11003.

3 E. Haak, "6 Easy Ways to Improve Your Memory," May 2013, oprah.com/health /How-to-Improve-Your-Memory-Remember-Things-Better/1.

4 M. A. Beydoun et al., "Helicobacter pylori Seropositivity and Cognitive Performance among US Adults: Evidence from a Large National Survey," *Psychosomatic Medicine* 75, no. 5 (June 2013): 486–96, ncbi.nlm.nih.gov/pubmed/23697465.

5 C. Roubaud Baudron et al., "Extragastric Diseases and *Helicobacter pylori*," *Helicobacter* 18, sup. 1 (September 2013): 44–51, ncbi.nlm.nih.gov/pubmed/24011245.

6 Julia Tolliver Maranan, "The Right Nutrients to Age-Proof Your Brain," *Natural Health* 33, no. 3 (April 2003): 64.

7 Genevieve Des Jarlais, "Alternatives to Prozac," AlternativeMedicine.com.

8 American Psychological Association, "Low Vitamin B$_{12}$ Is Associated with Poorer Memory in Older People with High Risk for Alzheimer's," *ScienceDaily* April 5, 2004, sciencedaily.com/releases/2004/04/040405085355.htm.

9 Ibid.

10 *"Helicobacter pylori* Tests," WebMD, webmd.com/digestive-disorders/helicobacter -pylori-tests.

11 "What Is Peptic Ulcer Disease?" WebMD, webmd.com/digestive-disorders/digestive -diseases-peptic-ulcer-disease.

12 E. P. Iakovenko et al., "Effects of Probiotic Bifiform on Efficacy of *Helicobacter pylori* Infection Treatment," *Terapevticheskii rkhiv* 78, no. 2 (2006): 21–26, ncbi.nlm.nih.gov/ pubmed/16613091.

13 Ibid.

14 "Product Review: Probiotics for Adults, Children, and Pets," February 23, 2015, consumerlab.com/reviews/Probiotic_Supplements_Lactobacillus_acidophilus_ Bifidobacterium/probiotics/.

15 M. Gotteland et al., "Modulation of *Helicobacter pylori* Colonization with Cranberry Juice and *Lactobacillus johnsonii* la1 in Children," *Nutrition* 24, no. 5 (2008): 421–26, ncbi.nlm.nih.gov/pubmed/18343637.

16 Y. T. Lin et al., "Inhibition of *Helicobacter pylori* and Associated Urease by Oregano and Cranberry Phytochemical Synergies," *Applied and Environmental Microbiology* 71, no. 12 (December 2005): 8558–864, ncbi.nlm.nih.gov/pubmed/16332847.

17 R. O'Mahony et al., "Bactericidal and Anti-Adhesive Properties of Culinary and Medicinal Plants against *H. pylori*," *World Journal of Gastroenterology* 11, no. 47 (December 21, 2005): 7499–507, ncbi.nlm.nih.gov/pubmed/16437723.

18 Alan C. Logan, *The Brain Diet: The Connection between Nutrition, Mental Health, and Intelligence* (Nashville, TN: Cumberland House Publishing, 2006), 115.

19 E. Guilllemard et al., "Consumption of a Fermented Dairy Product Containing the Probiotic *Lactobacillus casei* DN114001 Reduces the Duration of Respiratory Infections in the Elderly in a Randomised Controlled Trial," *British Journal of Nutrition* 103, no. 1 (January 2010): 58–68, ncbi.nlm.nih.gov/pubmed/19747410.

20 "Product Review: Probiotics for Adults, Children and Pets," February 23, 2015, consumerlab.com/reviews/Probiotic_Supplements_Lactobacillus_acidophilus _Bifidobacterium/probiotics/.

21 P. Bercik et al., "Chronic Gastrointestinal Inflammation Induces Anxiety-Like Behavior and Alters Central Nervous System Biochemistry in Mice," *Gastroenterology* 139, no. 6 (December 2010): 2102–12, ncbi.nlm.nih.gov/pubmed/20600016.

22 J. Feher et al., "Role of Gastrointestinal Inflammations in the Development and Treatment of Depression," *Orvosi Hetilap* 152, no. 37 (September 2012): 1477–85, ncbi.nlm.nih.gov/pubmed/21893478.

23 M. Messaoudi et al., "Assessment of Psychotropic-like Properties of a Probiotic Formulation (*Lactobacillus helveticus* R0052 and *Bifidobacterium longum* R0175) in Rats and Human Subjects," *British Journal of Nutrition* 105, no. 5 (March 2011): 755–64, ncbi.nlm.nih.gov/pubmed/20974015.

24 M. K. Park et al., "*Lactobacillus plantarum* DK119 as a Probiotic Confers Protection against Influenza Virus by Modulating Innate Immunity," *PLoS One* 8, no. 10 (October 4, 2013): e75368, ncbi.nlm.nih.gov/pubmed/24124485.

25 T. Schmitz-Hübsch et al., "Qigong Exercise for the Symptoms of Parkinson's Disease: A Randomized, Controlled, Pilot Study," *Movement Disorders: Official Journal of the Movement Disorder Society* 21, no. 4 (April 2006): 543–48, ncbi.nlm.nih.gov/ pubmed/16229022.

26 D. J. Wassom et al., "Qigong Exercise May Improve Sleep Quality and Gait Performance in Parkinson's Disease: A Pilot Study," *International Journal of Neuroscience*, published electronically ahead of publication on October 22, 2014, ncbi.nlm.nih.gov/pubmed/25233147.

27 T. L. Yost and A. G. Taylor, "Qigong as a Novel Intervention for Service Members with Mild Traumatic Brain Injury," *Explore* (NY) 9, no. 3 (May–June 2013): 142–49, ncbi.nlm.nih.gov/pubmed/23643369.

28 "Brain Scans, Blood Tests Show Positive Effects of Meditation," *Health Behavior News Service* (August 14, 2003), newswise.com/articles/brain-scans-blood-tests-show-positive -effects-of-meditation.

29 T. Htut, "The Effects of Meditation on the Body," September 18, 1999.

30 D. J. Wang et al., "Cerebral Blood Flow Changes Associated with Different Meditation Practices and Perceived Depth of Meditation," *Psychiatry Research* 191, no. 1 (January 30, 2011): 60–67, ncbi.nlm.nih.gov/pubmed/21145215.

31 B. Pradhan and H. Nagendra, "Immediate Effect of Two Yoga-Based Relaxation Techniques on Attention in Children," *International Journal of Yoga* 3, no. 2 (July 2010): 67–69, ncbi.nlm.nih.gov/pubmed/21170232.

32 Michelle Schoffro Cook, DNM, DAc, CNC, *The 4-Week Ultimate Body Detox Plan* (Toronto: John Wiley & Sons Ltd., 2006).

33 S. N. Katterman, "Mindfulness Meditation As an Intervention for Binge-Eating, Emotional Eating, and Weight Loss: A Systematic Review," *Eating Behaviors* 15, no. 2 (April 2014): 197–204, ncbi.nlm.nih.gov/pubmed/24854804.

34 Kathleen Doheny, "Remember This: Exercise Boosts Your Brain Power," April 6, 2012, webmd.com/fitness-exercise/news/20120406/remember-this-exercise-boosts-your -brainpower.

35 Ibid.

36 S. M. Landau et al., "Association of Lifetime Cognitive Engagement and Low ß-Amyloid Deposition," *Archives of Neurology* 69, no. 5 (2012): 623–29, dx.doi. org/10.1001/archneurol.2011.2748.

37 A. Lundqvist, K. Grundstrom, et al., "Computerized Training of Working Memory in a Group of Patients Suffering from Acquired Brain Injury," *Brain Injury* 24, no. 10 (September 2010): 1173–83, dx.doi.org/10.3109/02699052.2010.498007.

38 G. E. Smith, P. Housen, et al., "A Cognitive Training Program Based on Principles of Brain Plasticity: Results from the Improvement in Memory with Plasticity-Based Adaptive Cognitive Training (IMPACT) Study," *Journal of the American Geriatric Society* 57, no. 4 (April 2009): 594–603, ncbi.nlm.nih.gov/pubmed/19220558.

39 Laura Donnelly, "Running Guards Against Dementia, Keeps the Brain's Memory Centre Young: Study," March 17, 2014, news.nationalpost.com/2014/03/17/running-guards-against-dementia-keeps-the-brains-memory-centre-young-study/#__federated=1.

40 I. Sample, "Start Running and Watch Your Brain Grow, Say Scientists," *Guardian*, January 18, 2010, theguardian.com/science/2010/jan/18/running-brain-memory-cell -growth.

41 Kelly Crowe and Terry Reith, "Doctors Writing Prescriptions to Get Patients Active," May 4, 2013, cbc.ca/news/health/doctors-writing-prescriptions-to-get-patients -active-1.1355824.

42 K. Hotting et al., "Long Term Effects of Physical Exercise on Verbal Learning and Memory in Middle-Aged Adults: Results of a One-Year Follow Up Study," *Brain Sciences* 2, no. 3 (August 27, 2012): 332–46, ncbi.nlm.nih.gov/pubmed/24961197.

43 Y. Geda et al., "Caloric Intake, Aging, and Mild Cognitive Impairment: A Population-Based Study," *American Academy of Neurology (AAN)*, February 13, 2012.

44 J. M. Brunstrom, "Mind over Platter: Pre-Meal Planning and the Control of Meal Size in Humans," *International Journal of Obesity* (London) 38, sup. 1 (July 2014): S9–S12, ncbi.nlm.nih.gov/pmc/articles/PMC4105578/.

45 O. Khazan, "We Eat about 92% of the Food on Our Plates," *Atlantic*, July 25, 2014, theatlantic.com/health/archive/2014/07/we-eat-92-percent-of-the-food-on-our-plates /375016/.

Chapter 6

1   E. Guillemard et al., "Consumption of a Fermented Dairy Product Containing the Probiotic *Lactobacillus casei* DN114001 Reduces the Duration of Respiratory Infections in the Elderly in a Randomised Controlled Trial," *British Journal of Nutrition* 103, no. 1 (January 2010): 58–68, cbi.nlm.nih.gov/pubmed/19747410.

2   Alan C. Logan, *The Brain Diet* (Nashville, TN: Cumberland House Publishing, 2006), 115.

3   M. Tamura et al., "Effects of Probiotics on Allergic Rhinitis Induced by Japanese Cedar Pollen: Randomized Double-Blind, Placebo-Controlled Clinical Trial," *International Archives of Allergy and Immunology* 143, no. 1 (December 2007): 75–82, ncbi.nlm.nih.gov/pubmed/17199093.

4   "Could Deficiency in B Vitamins Be the Key Factor Spiking the Rise in Dementia and Alzheimer's?" September 28, 2010, articles.mercola.com/sites/articles/archive /2010/09/28/high-doses-of-b-vitamins-can-reduce-brain-shrinkage-memory-loss.aspx.

5   M. C. Morris et al., "Dietary Niacin and the Risk of Incident Alzheimer's Disease and of Cognitive Decline," *Journal of Neurology, Neurosurgery, and Psychiatry* 75, no. 8 (August 2004): 1093–99, ncbi.nlm.nih.gov/pubmed/15258207.

6   "Tryptophan, Niacin Protect Against Alzheimer's," July 16, 2004, newmediaexplorer.org /sepp/2004/07/16/tryptophan_niacin_protect_against_alzheimers.htm.

7   "Drugs and Supplements: Niacin," Mayo Clinic, November 1, 2013, mayoclinic.org /drugs-supplements/niacin--niacinamide/evidence/hrb-20059838.

8   Julia Tolliver Maranan, "The Right Nutrients to Age-Proof Your Brain," *Natural Health* 33, no. 3 (April 2003): 64.

9   M. S. Morris et al., "Depression and Folate Status in the US Population," *Psychotherapy and Psychosomatics* 72, no. 2 (March–April 2003): 80–87.

10 Julia Tolliver Maranan, "The Right Nutrients to Age-Proof Your Brain," *Natural Health* 33, no. 3 (April 2003): 64.

11 Ibid.

12 Genevieve Des Jarlais, "Alternatives to Prozac," March 1, 2005, mail.alternativemedicine.com /article-display/8697/subTopicID/172/Brain-Food-The-Natural-Cure-for-Depression.

13 "Low Vitamin B12 Is Associated with Poorer Memory in Older People with High Risk Genotype for Alzheimer's," *Neuropsychology*, April 4, 2004, apa.org/news/press/releases /2004/04/cognitive-support.aspx.

14 Ibid.

15 Julia Tolliver Maranan, "The Right Nutrients to Age-Proof Your Brain," *Natural Health* 33, no. 3 (April 2003): 64.

16 C. W. Shults, "Coenzyme Q10 Slows Progression of Parkinsons," *Archives of Neurology* 59, no. 10 (2002): 1541–50.

17 Ibid.

18 "Alzheimer's Linked to Mitochondrial Mutations," worldhealth.net/list/news /mitochondria/?page-11.

19 "Autism," *Alive Magazine*, alive.com.

20 Julia Tolliver Maranan, "The Right Nutrients to Age-Proof Your Brain," *Natural Health* 33, no. 3 (April 2003): 64.

21 Rachael Moeller Gorman, "Food for Thought: Can Healthy Eating Help Your Brain Stay Sharp?" *Eating Well*, April/May 2006.

22 Julia Tolliver Maranan, "The Right Nutrients to Age-Proof Your Brain," *Natural Health* 33, no. 3 (April 2003): 64.

23 Ibid.

24 A. G. Schulman et al., "Increased Risk of Parkinson's Disease after Depression: A Retrospective Cohort Study," *Neurology* 58 (2002): 1501–4.

25 H. M. van Praag, "Serotonin Precursors in the Treatment of Depression," *Advances in Biochemical Psychopharmacology* 34 (1982): 259–86, ncbi.nlm.nih.gov/ pubmed/6753514.

26 H. M. van Praag, "Management of Depression with Serotonin Precursors," *Biological Psychiatry* 16, no. 3 (March 1981): 291–310, ncbi.nlm.nih.gov/pubmed/6164407.

27 A. Soulairac and H. Lambinet, "Effect of 5-hydroxytryptophan, a Serotonin Precursor, on Sleep Disorders," *Annals of Medical Psychology* 1 (1977): 792–98.

28 I. Caruso, P. S. Puttini, M. Cazzola, and V. Azzolini, "Double-Blind Study of 5-hydroxytryptophan versus Placebo in the Treatment of Primary Fibromyalgia Syndrome," *Journal of International Medical Research* 18 (1990): 201–9.

29 Michael Murray, ND, *Dr. Murray's Total Body Tune-Up* (New York: Bantam Books, 2000).

30 James A. Duke, PhD, *Dr. Duke's Essential Herbs* (New York: St. Martin's Paperbacks, 2001), 140.

31 James Balch, MD, and Mark Stengler, ND, *Prescription for Natural Cures* (Hoboken, NJ: John Wiley & Sons, Inc., 2004), 37.

32 James A. Duke, PhD, *Dr. Duke's Essential Herbs* (New York: St. Martin's Paperbacks, 2001), 145.

33 Ibid., 144.

34 Ibid., 145.

35 Ibid., 141.

36 G. D'Andrea et al., "Herbal Therapy in Migraine," *Neurological Sciences* 35, sup. 1 (May 2014): 135–40, ncbi.nlm.nih.gov/pubmed/24867850.

37 J. Raghu et al., "The Ameliorative Effect of Ascorbic Acid and Ginkgo on Learning and Memory Deficits Associated with Fluoride Exposure," *Interdisciplinary Toxicology* 6, no. 4 (December 2013): 217–21, ncbi.nlm.nih.gov/pubmed/24678261.

38 James A. Duke, PhD, *Dr. Duke's Essential Herbs* (New York: St. Martin's Paperbacks, 2001), 153.

39 Julia Tolliver Maranan, "The Right Nutrients to Age-Proof Your Brain," *Natural Health* 33, no. 3 (April 2003): 64.

40 Ibid.

41 Ibid.

42 Mildred S. Seelig, MD, MPH, and Andrea Rosanoff, PhD, *The Magnesium Factor* (New York: Avery, 2003), 278.

43 Ibid.

44 Maria Noel Mandile, "Vinpocetine," *Natural Health*, January/February 2002.

45 Ibid.

46 Ibid.

47 David Perlmutter, MD, *BrainRecovery.com: Powerful Therapy for Challenging Brain Disorders* (Naples, FL: The Perlmutter Health Center, 2000), 6.

48 Ibid.

49 Ibid.

50 Lester Packer, PhD, and Carol Colman, *The Antioxidant Miracle* (New York: John Wiley & Sons, 1999), 19.

51 G. H. Marracci, R. E. Jones, G. P. McKeon, and D. N. Bourdette, "Alpha Lipoic Acid Inhibits T Cell Migration into the Spinal Cord and Suppresses and Treats Experimental Autoimmune Encephalomyelitis," *Journal of Neuroimmunology* 131,

no. 1–2 (2002): 104–114, ncbi.nlm.nih.gov/pubmed/12458042; M. Morini, L. Roccatagliata, R. Dell'Eva, et al., "Alpha-Lipoic Acid Is Effective in Prevention and Treatment of Experimental Autoimmune Encephalomyelitis," *Journal of Neuroimmunology* 148, no. 1–2 (2004): 146–53, ncbi.nlm.nih.gov/pubmed/14975595.

52 Lester Packer, PhD, and Carol Colman, *The Antioxidant Miracle* (New York: John Wiley & Sons, 1999), 157.

53 "Sage May Help Alzheimer's Sufferers," *Independent*, August 29, 2003, independent.co.uk.

54 P. J. Houghton, "Activity and Constituents of Sage Relevant to the Potential Treatment of Symptoms of Alzheimer's Disease," *Herbalgram: The Journal of the American Botanical Council* 61 (2004): 38–53.

55 "Sage May Help Alzheimer's Sufferers," *Independent* (August 29, 2003), independent.co.uk.

56 P. J. Houghton, "Activity and Constituents of Sage Relevant to the Potential Treatment of Symptoms of Alzheimer's Disease," *Herbalgram: The Journal of the American Botanical Council* 61 (2004): 38–53.

57 M. Nikfarjam et al., "The Effects of *Lavandula Angustifolia* Mill Infusion on Depression in Patients Using Citalopram: A Comparison Study," *Iranian Red Crescent Medical Journal* 15, no. 8 (August 2013): 734–39, ncbi.nlm.nih.gov/pubmed/24578844.

58 J. A. Duke, *Dr. Duke's Essential Herbs* (New York: St. Martin's Paperbacks, 2001), 359.

59 T. Matsumoto et al., "Does Lavender Aromatherapy Alleviate Premenstrual Emotional Symptoms? A Randomized Crossover Trial," *BioPsychoSocial Medicine* 7 (May 31, 2013): 12, ncbi.nlm.nih.gov/pubmed/23724853.

60 Rachael Moeller Gorman, "Food for Thought: Can Healthy Eating Help Your Brain Stay Sharp?" *Eating Well*, April/May 2006.

61 "Curry Ingredient May Stop Alzheimer's," *Medical News Today*, September 9, 2004, medicalnewstoday.com/medicalnews.php?newsid=13116.

62 P. Wang et al., "Mechanisms and Effects of Curcumin on Spatial Learning and Memory Improvement in APPswe/PS1dE9 Mice," *Journal of Neuroscience Research* 92, no. 2 (February 2014): 218–31, ncbi.nlm.nih.gov/pubmed/24273069.

63 N. Hishikawa et al., "Effect of Turmeric on Alzheimer's Disease with Behavioral and Psychological Symptoms of Dementia," *Ayu* 33, no. 4 (October 2012): 499–504, ncbi.nlm.nih.gov/pubmed/23723666.

64 A. M . Neyrinck et al., "*Curcuma longa* Extract Associated with White Pepper Lessens High Fat Diet-Induced Inflammation in Subcutaneous Adipose Tissue," *PLoS One* 8, no. 11 (November 12, 2013): e81252, ncbi.nlm.nih.gov/pubmed/24260564.

65 James Hamblin, "This is Your Brain on Fish," *Atlantic*, August 7, 2014, theatlantic.com /health/archive/2014/08/this-is-your-brain-on-fish/375638/.

66 James Balch, MD, and Mark Stengler, ND, *Prescription for Natural Cures* (Hoboken, NJ: John Wiley & Sons, Inc., 2004), 36.

67 Tolliver Maranan, "The Right Nutrients to Age-Proof Your Brain," *Natural Health*, April 2003.

68 Joseph Mercola, MD, "Keep Alzheimer's Away with Fish Oil's Secret Weapon," April 6, 2005, mercola.com.

69 "NINDS Neurotoxicity Information Page," National Institute of Neurological Disorders and Stroke, accessed August 16, 2013, ninds.nih.gov/disorders/neurotoxicity/neurotoxicity.htm.

70 *Biochimica et Biophysica Acta* 1792, no. 5 (May 2009): 432–43.

71 *Dialogues in Clinical Neurosciences* 15, no. 1 (March 2013): 67–76.

72 Ibid.

73 *Neurochemistry International* 60, no. 8 (June 2012): 827–36; *International Journal of Biochemistry and Molecular Biology* 3, no. 2 (2012): 219–41; Shou-Long Lu et al., "The Development of Nao Li Shen and its Clinical Application," *Journal of Pharmacy and Pharmacology* 49, no. 11 (1997): 1162–64; *Journal of Traditional Chinese Medicine* 17, no. 4 (December 1997): 299–303.

74 X. L. Wang et al., "Gastrodin Prevents Motor Deficits and Oxidative Stress in the MPTP Mouse Model of Parkinson's Disease: Involvement of ERK 1/2Nrf2 Signalling Pathway," *Life Sciences* 114, no. 2 (October 2, 2014): 77–85, ncbi.nlm.nih.gov /pubmed/25132361.

75 bbc.co.uk on the 11th June 2003.

76 *Journal of Pharmacy and Pharmacology* 49, no. 11 (November 1997): 1162–64 and *Journal of Traditional Chinese Medicine* 17, no. 4 (December 1997): 299–303.

77 Zhongguo Zhong Yao Za Zhi 9, no. 11 (November 2004): 1061–65; H. J. Kim, I. K. Hwang, and M. H. Won, "Vanillin, 4-hydroxybenzyl aldehyde and 4-hydroxybenzyl Alcohol Prevent Hippocampal CA1 Cell Death Following Global Ischemia," *Brain Research* 1181 (November 21, 2007): 130–41; S. J. An et al., "Gastrodin Decreases Immunoreactivities of Gamma-Aminobutyric Acid Shunt Enzymes in the Hippocampus of Seizure-Sensitive Gerbils," *Journal of Neuroscience Research* 71, no. 4 (February 15, 2003): 534–43.

78 *Journal of Ethnopharmacology* 56, no. 1 (March 1997): 45–54.

79 *Biological and Pharmaceutical Bulletin* 29, no. 2 (February 2006): 261–65; *China Clinical Practical Medicine* 5, no. 23 (August 2010): 160–61.

80 Z. L. Cai et al., "Effects of Cordycepin on Y-Maze Learning Task in Mice," *European Journal of Pharmacology* 714, no. 1–3 (August 2013): 249–53, ncbi.nlm.nih.gov /pubmed/23819912.

81 Z. Li et al., "*Cordyceps militaris* Extract Attenuates D-Galactose-Induced Memory Impairment in Mice," *Journal of Medicinal Food* 15, no. 12 (December, 2012): 1057–63, ncbi.nlm.nih.gov/pubmed/23216110.

82 J. Wang et al., "Anti-Inflammation and Antioxidant Effect of Cordymin, a Peptide Purified from the Medicinal Mushroom *Cordyceps silnensis*, in Middle Cerebral Artery Occlusion-Induced Focal Cerebral Ischemia in Rats," *Metabolic Brain Disease* 27, no. 2 (June 2012): 159–65, ncbi.nlm.nih.gov/pubmed/22327557.

83 Z. Cheng et al., "Cordycepin Protects against Cerebral Ischemia/Reperfusion Injury in vivo and in vitro," *European Journal of Pharmacology* 664, no. 1–3 (August 2011): 20–28, ncbi.nlm.nih.gov/pubmed/21554870.

84 Ibid.

85 J. Cho et al., "Antioxidant and Memory Enhancing Effects of Purple Sweet Potato Anthocyanin and Cordyceps Mushroom Extract," *Archives of Pharmacal Research* 26, no. 10 (October 2003): 821–25, ncbi.nlm.nih.gov/pubmed/14609130.

86 I. Tello et al., "Anticonvulsant and Neuroprotective Effects of Oligosaccharides from Lingzhi or Reishi Medicinal Mushroom, *Ganoderma lucidum* (Higher Basidiomycetes)," *International Journal of Medicinal Mushrooms* 15, no. 6 (2013): 555–68, ncbi.nlm.nih.gov/pubmed/24266379.

87 L. W. Chen et al., "Activating Mitochondrial Regulator PGC-1 Expression by Astrocytic NGF is a Therapeutic Strategy for Huntington's Disease," *Neuropharmacology* 63, no. 4 (September 2012): 719–32, ncbi.nlm.nih.gov/pubmed/22633948.

88 Ibid.

89 Z. Y. Zhou et al., "Neuroprotective Effects of Water-Soluble *Ganoderma lucidum* Polysaccharides on Cerebral Ischemic Injury in Rats," *Journal of Ethnopharmacology* 131, no. 1 (August 2010): 154–64, ncbi.nlm.nih.gov/pubmed/20600765.

INDEX

Underscored page references indicate boxed text.

A

Acetaldehyde, 68
Acetone, 77
Acetonitrile, 68
Acetylcholine
  acetylcholinesterase and, 186
  apples and, 103
  niacin and, 166–67
  rosemary and, 115
  thiamin and, 101
  vitamin B_{12} and, 168
Acetylcholinesterase (AChE), 186
Additives containing MSG, 55
Adenosine triphosphate (ATP), 182
Adrenal glands, 138
Aflatoxins, 100
Aged garlic extract (AGE), 125
Air fresheners, 71, 74–78
Alcohol
  brain disease and, 118
  hangovers after, 52
  in Standard American Diet,
    29–30
Allergies, 86, 165
Almonds
  Almond Milk, 223
  Apple and Almond Medley, 297
  Chocolate Truffles, 293
  Coco-Almond Butter, 218
  Dairy-Free Pasta Alfredo with
    Asparagus, 274
  Dairy-Free Vanilla Ice Cream, 292

fiber in, 100
as snack, 139
Alpha lipoic acid, 112, 182–85
Alpha-Terpineol, 69, 73
ALS, 15
Aluminum, 62, 65–67
Alzheimer's disease
  acetylcholine levels and, 186
  aluminum and, 66
  challenging brain, importance of,
    132–33
  copper and, 63
  game/puzzle playing and risk for,
    151, 153
  general discussion, 7
  H. pylori infections and, 134
  inflammation and, 7, 18, 94, 105,
    189
  MSG and, 54
  prescription medications and, 34–35
  saturated fat and, 36
  treatment options
    apples, 103
    coenzyme Q10, 171
    coffee, 119
    curcumin, 95, 189–91
    exercise, 153
    fish oil, 192
    folate, 167
    garlic, 125
    ginkgo biloba, 176
    niacin, 166
    pomegranates, 84

Alzheimer's disease (cont.)
  treatment options (cont.)
    resveratrol, 118
    sage, 89, 185, 186
    vitamin B$_{12}$, 168
    vitamin E, 172, 173
    walnuts, 109
  vitamin B$_{12}$ deficiency and, 42
Amaranth, 39
American diet. See Standard American Diet
Amino acids, 36–37
Amyloid plaques. See Plaques
Amyloid protein, 192
Amyotrophic lateral sclerosis (ALS), 15
Antacids, 65–67
Antibiotics, 135
Antidepressants, 188. See also Depression
Anti-inflammatories. See also Inflammation
  blueberries, 91
  caffeine, 119
  celery, 92–93
  cherries, 88, 89
  curcumin, 94, 96, 189–90
  garlic, 125
  ginger, 105–6
  NSAIDs, 106, 134–35
  olives, 113
  omega-6 fatty acids, 108–9
  onions, 124, 125
  probiotics, 165
  rosemary, 115
  sage, 187
Antioxidants
  alpha lipoic acid, 182–85
  in blueberries, 91
  in cherries, 87–88
  cordyceps, 195–96

  in ginkgo biloba, 176
  in olives, 112–13, 114
  in pitted fruits, 123
  in pomegranates, 84
  probiotics, 141, 162, 164
  resveratrol, 117–19
  in tea, 96–97, 98
  in tomatoes, 116
  vitamin E, 172–73
  in walnuts, 109
Anxiety
  curcumin and, 95, 190–91
  lavender and, 187
  probiotics and, 142
Aphrodisiac, ginkgo biloba as, 178
Apoptosis, 92, 166
Apple cider vinegar, 104, 105
Apples
  Apple and Almond Medley, 297
  Apple-Cinnamon-Walnut Oats, 216
  Curried Sweet Potato and Apple Soup, 242
  general discussion, 103–5
  Green Goddess Juice, 227
Arthritis
  celery for, 93
  cherries for, 89
  curcumin vs. drugs for, 94, 189–90
  dairy products and, 32–33
Artificial dyes, 71
Artificial sweeteners. See Sweeteners
Ascorbic acid (vitamin C)
  flavonoids and, 111
  gingko biloba and, 178
  inflammation and, 124
  when coping with stress, 140
Aspartame, 41, 51–53, 122
Atherosclerosis, 115, 116
ATP, 182

Attention
  games/puzzles and, 151
  meditation as improving, 146–47
  stretching as improving, 149
Avocado
  Avo-Salsa, 228, 231
  Chicken Summer Rolls, 287
  Guacamole, 229
  as source of protein, 37, 61
  Strawberry-Blueberry Pudding, 291
  Strawberry-Chocolate Royale, 298
Axons, 14, 131

B

Baby food, MSG in, 56
Bacteria. *See also* Probiotics
  friendly, 163
  gut–brain axis, 141–43
Baking soda
  as alternative to antacids, 66
  replacing fabric softener with, 71, 74
Bath products, toxic ingredients in, 71–72
B-complex vitamins. *See* Vitamin-B complex
BDNF, 49
Beans. *See also* Black beans; Chickpeas; Kidney beans
  general discussion, 101–2
  as source of fiber, 99
Bean sprouts
  Citrus-Ginger Salad, 250–51
  as source of protein, 37
  Thai Noodle Salad, 252–53
Beauty products, toxic ingredients in, 71–72
Bedtime, importance of set, 130
Benzodiazepines (BZDs), 34–35

Benzyl acetate, 69, 73
Benzyl alcohol, 69–70, 73
Berries. *See also* Blueberries; Strawberries
  cranberry juice, 136
  as source of fiber, 100
  Superbrainiac Breakfast Smoothie, 212
Beta amyloid, 95, 118, 151, 190
BHA, 71
BHT, 71
Bifidobacteria probiotic family
  effects on brain, 142
  gut health and, 163–64, 165
  for *H. pylori* infection, 135
Biotin, 184
Black beans
  fiber in, 99
  levels of vitamin B$_6$ and folate in, 101
  Warm Black Bean Salad, 246
  Wild Rice Salad with Corn and Beans, 255
Black tea, 96–98
Blenders, 207–8
Blood–brain barrier
  alpha lipoic acid and, 183
  chemicals in fragrances and, 69
  copper's effect on, 63
  mercury's ability to cross, 64
  MSG and, 54
  permeability of, 20
  trans fats as damaging, 25, 58
Blood flow
  gastrodin and, 194
  gingko biloba and, 175, 177
  meditation and, 146
  periwinkle and, 181
  rosemary and, 114
Blood pressure, 85, 124, 179

Blood sugar
  beans and, 102
  curcumin and, 191
  fiber and, 99
  stable levels of, 40, 139, 209
  tea drinking and, 97
Blueberries
  Blueberry Pancakes, 210
  general discussion, 90–92
  Green Tea and Blueberry Smoothie,
    214
  Grilled Salmon with Plum-
    Blueberry-Grape Salsa,
    279
  Salade de Provence, 247
  Strawberry-Blueberry Pudding,
    292
Bok choy, 238
Bottled sauces, MSG in, 56
Brain. *See also* 4-Week Brain Health
    Challenge; *specific brain-
    boosting tips*
  author's research on, 5–6
  challenging, importance of,
    131–33
  control over capacity and health of,
    4
  general discussion, 3–5
  gut–brain axis, 141–43, 162–63
  of infants, capacity of, 15–16
  power of, 14–16
  shrinkage, 153, 166
  transforming, 19–21
Brain Books in Action, 79–80, 126,
    158
Brain-boosting superfoods, 41, 81–83.
    See also specific superfoods
Brain cancer, 196
Brain-derived neurotrophic factor
    (BDNF), 49

Brain disease. *See also specific diseases*
  deaths caused by, 20
  link between inflammation and,
    16–19
  link to prescription medications,
    34–35
  probiotics and, 162, 164
  program usefulness in cases of, 6, 8
  risk of, 10–13
Brain health assessment, 6, 10–13
Brain Health Plan. *See* 4-Week Brain
    Health Challenge
Brain injury
  games/puzzles and, 151
  overview, 5–6
  pomegranate consumption and,
    84–85
  qigong and, 144
  signs of, 8–9
Brain Power in Action Success Tips, 199
Breast cancer, 87
Brown rice
  Curried Chickpeas and Rice, 270
  Dairy-Free Pasta Alfredo with
    Asparagus, 274
  overview, 39
  Pineapple-Basil Rice, 269
  Red Lentil and Rice Soup, 235
  Rice Salad with Curried Tofu,
    254
  Southwestern Bruschetta, 228
Buckwheat
  Chicken Pho with Buckwheat
    Noodles, 238
  Chicken Summer Rolls, 287
  fiber in, 100
Butane, 77
Butylated hydroxyanisole (BHA), 71
Butylated hydroxytoluene (BHT), 71
BZDs, 34–35

C

Cadmium, 62–63, 65
Caffeine. *See also* Coffee; Tea
  age-related degenerative process
      and, 97
  calculating intake, 120
  health benefits of, 123
  inflammation and, 119
  when to avoid, 120
Cancer
  blueberries and, 92
  coffee and, 123
  cordyceps and, 196–97
  pomegranates and, 87
  resveratrol and, 119
  rosemary and, 115–16
  tomatoes and, 117
Carbohydrates
  in 4-Week Brain Health Challenge,
      37–39
  in Standard American Diet,
      27–29
Carnosic acid, 115–16
Carrots
  Roasted Carrot Soup, 236
Carter, Renee, 126, 199
Catechins, 96
Celery
  general discussion, 92–93
  Green Goddess Juice, 227
Celiac disease, 39
Celtic sea salt, 42
Centrifugal juicers, 207
Cervac, Donna, 79–80, 199
Challenges, importance to brain
      health, 131–33
Chemical scents, 67–72
Cherries
  general discussion, 87–89, 123

Orange and Dried Cherry Porridge,
    215
Orange Balsamic Halibut with Mint
    and Dried Cherries, 281
Quinoa Salad with Cherries and
    Pecans, 256
Chickpeas
  adding to diet, 102
  Curried Chickpeas and Rice, 270
  fiber in, 99
  Hearty Chickpea Soup, 241
  Hummus, 233
  Moroccan Stuffed Peppers, 273
Chloroform, 70, 73
Chlorogenic acid, 105
Cholesterol
  apples and, 103–4, 105
  ginger and, 106
  olives and, 113
  onions and, 124
Choline, 177
Chromium, 124
Chronic fatigue syndrome, 182
Chronic inflammation, 17–18
Circulation, ginkgo biloba and, 176,
    178
Citrus juicers, 207
Coal tar, 71
Coconut oil
  Brain-Boosting Butter, 230
  Coco-Almond Butter, 218
  overview, 41
Coconut sugar, 121
Coenzyme Q10 (CoQ10), 170–72
Coffee
  general discussion, 119–23
  Super-Health-Boosting Pumpkin
      Spice "Latte", 224–25
Colognes, 67–68, 70–71
Concussions, 8–9

Copper, 63–64
CoQ10, 170–72
Cordyceps, 195–97
COX-1, 94, 190
COX-2, 94, 190
COX-2 inhibitors, 94, 190
Cranberry juice, 136
C-reactive protein, 17, 18, 60
Creamers, coffee, 122
Croutons, MSG in, 56
Curcumin. *See also* Curry
  in general brain health plan, 43
  general discussion, 94–96,
    189–91
  for *H. pylori infections*, 136
Curry. *See also* Curcumin
  Coconut Curried Tofu with
    Macadamia Nuts, 268
  Curried Cauliflower, 278
  Curried Chickpeas and Rice,
    270
  Curried Sweet Potato and Apple
    Soup, 242
  Rice Salad with Curried Tofu, 254
  Shrimp in Green Tea-Curry Sauce,
    286
Cycling, 148–50
Cyclooxygenase, 125
Cyclooxygenase-1 (COX-1), 94, 190
Cyclooxygenase-2 (COX-2), 94, 190
Cytokines, 163

D

Dairy products
  alternatives to, 61, 122
  in coffee, 122
  in 4-Week Brain Health Challenge,
    36–37
  in Standard American Diet, 31–33

Dandelion root
  Super-Health-Boosting Pumpkin
    Spice "Latte", 224–25
DBP, 71
DEA, 71
Dehydration, 140
Dementia. *See also* Alzheimer's disease
  gastrodin and, 194
  H. pylori infections and, 134
  intellectual games and, 153
  niacin and, 167
  periwinkle and, 181
  vitamin E and, 173
  walking and, 152, 153
Deodorizers, 71, 74–78
Depression
  general discussion, 17
  gluten sensitivity and, 39–40
  link to intestinal inflammation, 142
  treatment options
    5-HTP, 173–74, 175
    folate, 167
    lavender, 187–88
    probiotics, 142
    vitamin B_{12}, 168
  vitamin B_{12} deficiency and, 42
DHA, 107–8, 192–93
Diabetes, 120
Dibutyl phthalate (DBP), 71
Diet foods/beverages, 51–53
Diethanolamine (DEA), 71
Digestive health, 141–43, 162–63
Dihydrotestosterone, 115
DNA, 86–87, 90
Docosahexaenoic acid (DHA), 107–8,
  192–93
Dopamine, 52, 91, 97
Dried fruits, 123–24
Dryer sheets, 73–74
Dyes, 71
Dysthymia, 167

E

Education, relation to brain health, 132

EGCG, 97

Eicosapentaenoic acid (EPA), 193

Ellagic acid, 92

Energy
   in brain cells, periwinkle and, 182
   coenzyme Q10 and, 170, 171, 172
   spinach and, 112

Enriched-flour products, 38

Enzymes, 65

EPA, 193

Epigallocatechin gallate (EGCG), 97

Equipment, kitchen, 205–6

Essential oils
   for fragrance, 70–71
   fragrance oils vs., 69
   lavender, 140, 188

Ethanol, 70, 73

Ethyl acetate, 70, 74

Excitotoxins, 54–55

Exercise
   effects on brain, 152–54
   in 4-Week Brain Health Challenge, 42
   prescriptions for, 154
   stretching and cycling, 148–50
   tai chi and qigong, 143–45
   walking, 152–55

Extra-virgin olive oil, 26, 41, 113

F

Fabric softeners
   neurotoxins found in, 69–70, 73–74
   substituting, 71, 74

Fair trade coffee, 121

Farmed salmon, 108

Fats. *See also specific types of fat*
   in 4-Week Brain Health Challenge, 36–37, 40, 57–59
   in Standard American Diet, 25–27

Fatty acids. *See also* Omega-3 fatty acids
   omega-6, 25–26, 37, 107
   omega-9, 113

Fiber, 98–101

Field, Dawn, 199

Filtered water, 65

Fish
   containing omega-3 fatty acid, 108
   Grilled Salmon with Plum-Blueberry-Grape Salsa, 279
   mercury in, 108
   Orange Balsamic Halibut with Mint and Dried Cherries, 281
   Roast Cod with Pomegranate-Walnut Sauce, 280
   Toasted Millet Salad with Salmon, 282–83
   wild-caught, 30

Fish oil, 192–93

5-hydroxytryptophan (5-HTP), 173–75

Flavonoids (vitamin P)
   in blueberries, 90–91
   in cherries, 88
   in ginkgo biloba, 176
   in pitted fruits, 88, 123
   in spinach, 110–11

Flavored syrups, for coffee, 121–22

Flaxseed oil
   Brain-Boosting Butter, 230
   Coco-Almond Butter, 218
   heating, 26
   omega-3 fatty acids in, 107, 108

Flaxseeds
   Apple-Cinnamon-Walnut Oats, 216
   fiber in, 100
   omega-3 fatty acids in, 107, 108
   as source of protein, 61

Folate (vitamin B$_9$)
  in beans, 101, 102
  general discussion, 167
  supplementation with, 168–69
Food processors, 206
4-Week Brain Health Challenge
  brain health assessment, 10
  customizing, 24
  overview, 6, 8, 23–24
  principles of, 36–43
  60-Second Brain Health Tips, 43
Fragrance oils, 69
Fragrances, 67–72
Free radicals. *See also* Antioxidants
  alpha lipoic acid as attacking, 182,
    183, 184
  effects on brain, 172, 176
  ORAC scale, 84
  probiotics and, 141, 162, 164
  tea and, 96, 98
  vinpocetine's effect on, 181
Fresh air, when coping with stress, 140
Fried foods, 26–27
Fruit. *See also specific fruit*
  benefits of diet rich in, 60
  in 4-Week Brain Health Challenge,
    40–41
  as source of fiber, 99

Ginger Lemonade, 220
  Roasted Miso-Ginger Tofu, 266
Ginkgo biloba, 43, 175–78
Gluten
  inflammation caused by, 33–36,
    38
  mental illness and, 39–40
  sensitivity to, 38
Grains. *See also specific grains*; Whole
    grains
  in 4-Week Brain Health Challenge,
    37–39
  in Standard American Diet, 33–36
Grapes
  Grilled Salmon with Plum-
    Blueberry-Grape Salsa, 279
  Mediterranean Quinoa Salad, 260
  resveratrol in, 118
  Superbrainiac Breakfast Smoothie,
    212
Greens. *See* Leafy greens; Spinach
Green tea
  general discussion, 96–98
  Green Tea and Blueberry Smoothie,
    214
  Iced Pomegranate Green Tea,
    221
  Shrimp in Green Tea-Curry Sauce,
    286
Gut–brain axis, 141–43, 162–63

G

Games, 150–52, 153
Garbanzo beans. *See* Chickpeas
Garlic, 125
Gastrodin, 193–95
Gastrointestinal tract, 141–43, 162–63
Ginger
  Citrus-Ginger Salad, 250–51
  general discussion, 105–6

H

Hair regrowth, rosemary and, 115
Hangovers, 52
HD
  general discussion, 19
  reishi and, 197
Headaches, 178, 195

Heart disease
    apples and, 103–4, 105
    fish oil and, 193
    resveratrol and, 118
    tomatoes and, 116
    walnuts and, 110
Heart rate, calculating target, 150
Heat shock proteins (stress proteins),
        91
Heavy metals, 62–65
Helicobacter pylori (*H. pylori*)
        infections, 133–37
Herbs. *See specific herbs*
Hippocampus
    effects of Alzheimer's disease on,
        7
    exercise and, 149, 153
    fish oil and, 192
    phthalates and, 75
Homocysteine, 101, 124, 168, 169
Hormones. *See also* Neurotransmitters;
        specific hormones
    aspartame and, 52
    in dairy products, 32
    in poultry, 30
    scents and, 72
    stress, 138
Huntington's disease (HD)
    general discussion, 19
    reishi and, 197
Hydrogenated fats, 40, 107. *See also*
        Trans fats

I

Ice cream makers, 205–6
IL-6, 164
Immune response, inflammation in,
        17

Immunity
    alpha lipoic acid and, 185
    cordyceps and, 197
    digestive health and, 163
    game/puzzle playing and, 152
    kimchi as boosting, 143
    pomegranates and, 86
    reishi and, 198
    sugar consumption and, 51
Infant formula, MSG in, 56
Infants, brain capacity of, 15–16
Infection, pomegranates and, 86
Inflammation. *See also* Anti-
        inflammatories
    Alzheimer's disease and, 7, 105, 189
    brain diseases and, link between,
        16–19
    chronic, 17–18
    dairy products and, 32–33
    digestive health and, 163
    fats and, 25–27, 59, 107, 108–9
    foods causing, 31
    gluten and, 33–35, 38
    H. pylori infections producing, 134
    intestinal, link to depression, 142
    meat consumption and, 30, 59–61
    Parkinson's disease and, 105
    as predictor of brain health, 15
    Standard American Diet and,
        24–25
    sugar and, 28
Insomnia, 175, 188
Intellectual challenges, relation to
        brain health, 132–33
Intellectual games, dementia and, 153
Interleukin-6 (IL-6), 164
Intestines
    fiber's effects on, 98
    gut–brain axis, 141–43, 162–63
Intrinsic factor, 169

Iodized salt, 42
Isobutane, 77

J

Juicers, 206–7

K

Kidney beans
  fiber in, 99
  levels of vitamin B$_6$ and folate in, 101
  manganese in, 102
  Mediterranean Bean, Potato, and
    Vegetable Salad Platter, 248
Kidneys, pomegranate consumption
    and, 86
Kimchi, 143
Kitchen equipment, 205–8

L

Lactobacillus probiotic family
  effects on brain, 141–43
  gut health and, 163–65
  for *H. pylori* infection, 135, 136
Language skills, synapses related to,
    131–33
Laundry soap, 71
Lavender
  for coping with stress, 140
  essential oils, 140, 188
  general discussion, 187–89
  improving sleep with, 130, 188
  Salade de Provence, 247
Lead, sources of, 64, 72

Leafy greens. *See also* Spinach
  adding to diet, 111–12
  Basil-Lettuce-Tomato-Pepper
    (BLTP) Sandwiches, 264
  Citrus-Ginger Salad, 250–51
  health benefits of, 112
  Mediterranean Bean, Potato, and
    Vegetable Salad Platter,
    248
  Mediterranean Quinoa Salad,
    260
  Mixed Greens Salad with Fall Fruit
    and Beet Dressing, 261
  Roasted Sweet Potato Salad, 249
  Salade de Provence, 247
  as source of fiber, 101
  Thai Noodle Salad, 252–53
Learning, relation to brain health,
    132–33
Legumes. *See also specific legumes*
  in 4-Week Brain Health Challenge,
    41
  general discussion, 38, 101–2
  as source of fiber, 99
  as source of protein, 61
Lentils
  adding to diet, 102
  fiber in, 99
  Lentil Burgers, 263
  Red Lentil and Rice Soup, 235
  Savory Lentil Stew, 237
Lewis, Janine, 199
Linalool, 70, 74
Lipase, 193
Lipoxygenase, 125
Liquefied petroleum gas, 77
Liver health, 86, 124
Lou Gehrig's Disease, 15
Lycopene, 116, 117

M

Magnesium, 178–80
Mandel, Mitch, 199
Manganese, 102
Margarine, 25, 58–59
Masticating juicers, 207
MEA, 71
Meals
  1-Week Meal Plan, 299–302
  in 4-Week Brain Health Challenge,
    40
  skipping, 139
Meat
  in 4-Week Brain Health Challenge,
    36–37, 59–61
  inflammation caused by, 30, 59–61
  in Standard American Diet, 30
Medications, link to brain disease,
    34–35. *See also specific types of
    medication*
Meditation
  for coping with stress, 140
  effects on brain, 145–47
  health benefits of, 148
  practicing, 147–48
Memory
  challenging brain, importance for,
    131–33
  overeating and, 155–56
  protecting from damage, 4, 6, 20
  stress and, 138
  treatments to improve
    alpha lipoic acid, 183–84
    cordyceps, 196
    curcumin, 190
    games/puzzles, 151
    garlic, 125
    gingko biloba, 176

periwinkle, 180–81
rosemary, 114–15
sage, 185
sleep, 129
stretching and cycling, 148–49
trying something new, 137
vitamin B$_{12}$, 168
vitamin B$_{12}$ deficiency and, 42
Mental illness, gluten sensitivity and,
    39–40
Mercury, 64, 108
Metabolic syndrome, 53, 86
Migraines, 178
Milk
  in coffee, 122
  dairy alternatives, 61, 122
  in Standard American Diet, 31–33
Millet
  fiber in, 100
  Millet and Sweet Potato Cakes, 272
  Moroccan Stuffed Peppers, 273
  Orange and Dried Cherry Porridge,
    215
  Spice-Rubbed Chicken with Millet
    Pilaf, 289
  Toasted Millet Salad with Salmon,
    282–83
Mineral supplements, 42–43
Mini-mental state examination
    (MMSE), 95, 191
Miso
  Miso Soup, 239
  Roasted Miso-Ginger Tofu, 266
  as source of protein, 61
Mitochondria
  coenzyme Q10 and, 170, 171
  docosahexaenoic acid and, 108
  monounsaturated fats and, 112
MMSE, 95, 191

Monoethanolamine (MEA), 71
Monosodium glutamate (MSG)
    in additives, 55
    effects on brain, 53–55
    health benefits of avoiding, 57
    hidden sources of, 56–57
    in protein powders, 61
Monounsaturated fats, 112–13
Mood, improving
    5-HTP, 173–74
    lavender, 187
    sage, 185, 186
Motor neuron disease, 15
MSG
    in additives, 55
    effects on brain, 53–55
    health benefits of avoiding, 57
    hidden sources of, 56–57
    in protein powders, 61
Multiple sclerosis, 184
Multivitamin supplements, 42–43
Musk tetralin, 68
Myelin sheath, 40

N

Navy beans, 102
Neurons, 14–15
Neurotoxins. *See also specific*
        neurotoxins
    defined, 21
    in fabric softeners, 73–74
    in fragrances, 68–70
Neurotransmitters. *See also specific*
        neurotransmitters
    B-complex vitamins and, 166
    overview, 14–15
    synapses and, 131
    vitamin B_{12} and, 134, 168

New things, trying, 137–38
Niacin (vitamin B_3), 166–69
Niacinamide, 169
Nonsteroidal anti-inflammatory drugs
        (NSAIDs)
    ginger vs., 106
    H. pylori infections and, 134–35
Nutrition, relation to brain health, 16
Nuts. *See also* Almonds; Walnuts
    eating when traveling, 209
    as source of fiber, 99–100
    as source of protein, 61

O

Oats/oatmeal
    Apple-Cinnamon-Walnut Oats, 216
    fiber in, 100
    gluten in, 35
    Lentil Burgers, 263
    Quick Spelt Bread, 219
Obesity, diet soda and, 53
Oils
    essential, 69, 70–71, 140, 188
    in 4-Week Brain Health Challenge,
        41
    fragrance, 69
    smoke point of, 26–27, 113
    in Standard American Diet, 26–27
Olive oil, 26, 41, 113
Olives, 112–14
Omega-3 fatty acids
    fish oil, 192–93
    general discussion, 107–9
    heating, 230
    link between inflammation and
        depression, 142
    in Standard American Diet, 25–26
    trans fats and, 58

PMS, 188–89
Polyphenols, 109, 110–11, 113
Pomegranates
    Berry Special Chicken Salad, 262
    Broccoli Stem, Quinoa, and
        Edamame Salad, 258–59
    general discussion, 84–87
    Iced Pomegranate Green Tea, 221
    Mediterranean Quinoa Salad, 260
    Mixed Greens Salad with Fall Fruit
        and Beet Dressing, 261
    Pomegranate Lemonade, 222
    Pomegranate Salsa, 232
    Roast Cod with Pomegranate-
        Walnut Sauce, 280
    Walnut-Crusted Chicken Breasts
        with Pomegranate Syrup, 288
Portion sizes, 156–57
Potassium sorbate, 121
Poultry
    in 4-Week Brain Health Challenge,
        36–37
    in Standard American Diet, 30
Premenstrual syndrome (PMS),
    188–89
Prepared foods
    MSG in, 53, 56–57
    in Standard American Diet, 31
Prescription medications, link to brain
    disease, 34–35
Pritchard, Shelagh, 158
Proanthocyanidins, 88, 91, 123, 124
Probiotics. *See also specific probiotic
    strains*
    general discussion, 162–65
    gut–brain axis, 141–43
    health benefits of, 137, 143,
        164–65
    H. pylori infections, knocking out,
        135, 136

Processed foods
    MSG in, 53
    in Standard American Diet, 31
Propane, 77
Prostaglandins, 94, 190
Prostate cancer, 87
Protein
    in 4-Week Brain Health Challenge,
        36–37
    plant-based sources of, 37, 61
Protein powder, MSG in, 56, 61
Psychosis, gluten sensitivity and, 39
Puzzles, 150–53

Q

Qigong, 144–45
Quercetin, 124
Quinoa
    Broccoli Stem, Quinoa, and
        Edamame Salad, 258–59
    Greek Quinoa Toss, 271
    Mediterranean Quinoa Salad, 260
    overview, 39
    Protein-Rich Quinoa Salad, 257
    Quinoa Salad with Cherries and
        Pecans, 256
    Seared Sea Scallops with Quinoa
        Pilaf, 284–85

R

Red wine, resveratrol in, 118
Refined grains, 37, 38
Reishi mushrooms, 197–98
Relaxation
    coping with stress through, 140
    for improving sleep, 130

Restaurants, eating well at, 208
Resveratrol, 30, 43, 117–19
Rice. *See* Brown rice; Wild rice
Rosemary, 114–16

S

Saccharin, 41, 122
Saccharomyces probiotics, 135, 136
Sage, 89–90, 185–87
St. John's wort, 174
Salad dressings, 56, 245
Salads. *See also specific recipes by brain-boosting superfood*
brain-boosting ingredients for, 243–44
eating at restaurants, 208
Salad spinners, 205
Salicylic acid, 91
Salmon
farmed, 108
Grilled Salmon with Plum-Blueberry-Grape Salsa, 279
Toasted Millet Salad with Salmon, 282–83
Salt, 42
Saturated fats, 36, 37. *See also* Trans fats
Sauces, MSG in bottled, 56
Scents, chemical, 67–72
Schizophrenia, gluten sensitivity and, 39
Sea salt, 42
Seeds
eating when traveling, 209
as snack, 139
as source of fiber, 100
as source of protein, 61
Sensory environment, relation to brain health, 16

Serotonin, 52, 174
Sesame seeds
fiber in, 100
Stir-Fried Asparagus with Sesame Seeds, 277
Shortening, 25
Skin cancer, 87
Skin-care products, toxic ingredients in, 71–72
Skin health, vitamin E and, 173
Skipping meals, 139
Sleep
5-HTP and, 175
general discussion, 129–31
lavender as improving, 130, 188
Slowing down, importance of, 139
Smoke points, oil, 26–27, 113
Snacks, 40
SOD, 102, 196
Soda
diet, 51–53
as source of sugar, 50
Sodium benzoate, 121
Sodium lauryl sulfate, 72
Soups, MSG in, 56
Soy products, 56–57, 61. *See also* Tofu
Spelt
as gluten-containing, 35, 38
Quick Spelt Bread, 219
Southwestern Bruschetta, 228
Spice mixtures, MSG in, 57
Spinach
Berry Special Chicken Salad, 262
Chicken Summer Rolls, 287
general discussion, 110–12
Greek Quinoa Toss, 271
Split peas
Slow-Cooker Split Pea Soup, 240
Squash, as source of fiber, 101

Standard American Diet
  alcohol, 29–30
  carbohydrates, 27–29
  fats, 25–27, 107
  grains, 33–36
  meat and poultry, 30
  milk and dairy, 31–33
  overview, 24–25
  processed, packaged, and prepared
      foods, 31
  sweeteners, 30
Statin drugs, 103–4
Stearalkonium chloride, 72
Stevia
  in coffee, 121
  general discussion, 50–51
  Ginger Lemonade, 220
  Pomegranate Lemonade, 222
  replacing aspartame with, 52–53
Strawberries
  Berry Special Chicken Salad, 262
  fiber in, 100
  polyphenols in, 111
  Soy Fruit Smoothie, 213
  Strawberry-Blueberry Pudding, 292
  Strawberry-Chocolate Royale, 298
  Strawberry Gelato, 296
  Water-Berry Juice, 226
Stress
  coping with, 139–40
  health benefits of dealing with, 140
  link between inflammation and, 18
  meditation and, 146
  reishi and, 198
  stress, 138–49
Stress proteins (heat shock proteins), 91
Stretching, 148–50
Stroke
  alpha lipoic acid and, 184
  apples and, 103–4

  cordyceps and, 196
  exercise and, 153
  gastrodin and, 194
  ginger and, 106
  magnesium and, 179
  onions and, 124
  periwinkle and, 181
  pomegranate and, 85
  reishi and, 197
  resveratrol and, 118
  tea and, 97
  tomatoes and, 116
Sucralose, 41, 122
Sugar
  body's need for, 37–38
  coconut, 121
  in coffee, 121
  danger of consuming, 49, 51
  in dried fruits, 123–24
  in 4-Week Brain Health Challenge,
      41–42
  hidden sources of, <u>28–29</u>
  in Standard American Diet, 27–28
  substituting, 49–51
Sugar-free syrups, in coffee, 122
Sulfites, 113, 123–24
Sulfur compounds, in onions, 124
Superfoods, 81–83. *See also specific
      superfoods*
Superoxide dismutase (SOD), 102, 196
Supplements, 42–43. *See also specific
      supplements*
Sweeteners
  aspartame, 51–53
  in coffee, 121, 122
  in 4-Week Brain Health Challenge,
      41
  general discussion, 30
  natural, 50
  stevia, 50–51

Sweet potatoes
  Curried Sweet Potato and Apple
    Soup, 242
  Millet and Sweet Potato Cakes, 272
  Roasted Sweet Potato Salad, 249
Synapses, 14, 131–32
Syrups, flavored, for coffee, 121–22

T

Tai chi, 143–45
Tea. *See also* Green tea
TEA, 71
Tea
  ensuring healthiness of, 121
  general discussion, 96–98
Terpenes, 176
Thiamin (vitamin B$_1$), 101
Tofu
  Brain-Building Eggless Scramble, 211
  Coconut Curried Tofu with
    Macadamia Nuts, 268
  Easy Tofu Stir-Fry for One, 267
  Roasted Hoisin Tofu, 265
  Roasted Miso-Ginger Tofu, 266
  as source of protein, 37, 61
Toluene, 68, 72
Tomatoes
  Basil-Lettuce-Tomato-Pepper
    (BLTP) Sandwiches, 264
  Brain-Building Salsa, 231
  general discussion, 116–17
  Greek Quinoa Toss, 271
  Green Bean Ragout, 275
  Smoky Grilled Chicken with
    Tomato Chutney, 290–91
Trans fats
  as bad fats, 25–26
  in coffee whiteners, 122

eliminating, 40
in Standard American Diet, 107
substituting, 57–59
Traumatic brain injury
  games/puzzles and, 151
  overview, 5–6
  pomegranate consumption and,
    84–85
  qigong and, 144
  signs of, 8–9
Traveling, eating well when, 208–9
Triclosan, 72
Triethanolamine (TEA), 71
Trying something new, 137–38
Turmeric. *See also* Curry
  Brain-Building Eggless Scramble, 211
  general discussion, 94–96, 189–91
  for *H. pylori infections*, 136

V

Vaccines, MSG in, 57
Vegetable oil, 26
Vegetables. *See also specific vegetables*
  benefits of diet rich in, 60
  crudités, 245
  in 4-Week Brain Health Challenge,
    40–41
  as source of fiber, 99
Vinegar
  apple cider, 104, 105
  replacing fabric softener with, 74
Vinpocetine, 180–82
Vision, improving, 112, 117
Vitamin A, 112
Vitamin B$_1$ (thiamin), 101
Vitamin B$_{12}$
  effects on brain, 166, 168
  H. pylori infections, effect of, 134